The Cannabis Guide

Reprogramming the Body & Mind for Wellness

Written by:

Jacob Titus St. James

Edited by:

Amy Brooks

Reviewed by:

Chingling Wo, Ph D.

Illustrated by:

Noelle Ho

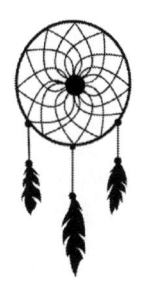

Table of Contents

Introduction……………………………………….7
Let's Talk About Getting High…………………..10
Mind-Body Interconnection…………….……….13
Dealing with Disease: Tools for Happiness……..21
The Endocannabinoid System…………………...32
Marijuana……………....……………..…………38
Cannabis………………..…..…………..….……46
Hemp……….……..….…..………….………...49
Entourage Effect & Whole Plant Medicine ….…..51
Plant cannabinoids……..…..………..…....……..58
Terpenes……….…....…..…………....………...60
Using Cannabis……………....……………..…...61
Biological Chemistry: Metabolism…….…......…..64
Choosing Products……..…..……..….…..……..66
Dosing Cannabis……………....…………..…….69
Methods of Consumption……………………….73
Growing Cannabis ……………...…………..…..83
Harvesting & Curing…………………………. 86
Crafting Cannabis………..……….…......…..….89
Simple Recipes………………...…..……………90
Cautions……………………………….......…...95
Journal…………………………………………...102

© Jacob St. James, 2019

Not intended to treat, cure, or diagnose medical conditions.
May not be reproduced without author consent. No copyright
infringement intended.

Welcome

As cannabis is now available recreationally and medicinally in many states, it's good to know how to use it. The information presented in these pages is simplified and meant to help build a basic understanding of how the body works, grows, and heals. This manual is a collection of research, experience, insights, and publicly available information to help answer the most commonly asked questions about cannabis. Many people walk into a medical marijuana store expecting the budtender, or person behind the counter, to answer all their questions about cannabis. Budtenders have limited education. They can answer some questions about the products they sell in-store, but everyone varies in their knowledge and experience. Budtenders are mostly trained by company salespersons that are in no way medical health professionals.

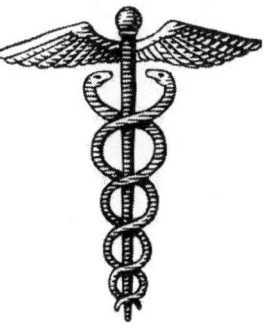

There is a flaw in separating conventional and alternative medicine. Western medicine tends to ignore the psychological, social, and environmental factors of disease. It overlooks the power of positive thinking, spirituality, and natural plant medicine. While herbs may not seem to be a part of Western medicine, all pharmaceuticals are made from plants.

The slitting of cannabis use into recreational and medicinal across the country is flawed. Cannabis is most often used *therapeutically* to relieve anxiety, reduce pain, increase happiness, and treat serious illness. It enhances the brain activity and allows users to feel more connected, aware, and present. Thousands of years of knowledge and evidence have been passed down through generations of healers that discovered the medicinal properties of cannabis plants. The love involved in nurturing, harvesting, preparing, and using plants for food and medicine is what connects people to each other and the earth. Modern medicine has been rediscovering the health benefits of cannabis after decades of stigma and prohibition. Cannabis inspires *renaissance*—not revolution.

Cannabis is an entheogen; a drug that helps a person become inspired and *come into being*. It has been used for centuries to achieve enlightenment, unravel mysteries of the subconscious, enhance mind-body awareness, as an aphrodisiac, and as powerful medicine. Cannabis works to balance hormones, is a powerful anti-inflammatory, and pain-killer.

Cannabis is safe, non-toxic, non-addictive and one of many tools for well-being that can be integrated into a healthy lifestyle with conscious consumption and responsible use. Balanced diet, enjoyable exercise, and relaxation techniques enhance the medicinal benefits, effects, and absorption of plant medicine. Plants and herbs can be used as part of holistic therapy to heal from or prevent disease.

Plant medicines aren't designed to cure us. They help us recognize our truth and lead us towards the next steps we have to take to heal. Cannabis is a bridge to healthy living. The ultimate goal is learning to practice self-care. Positive thinking, relaxation techniques, and activities that spark joy keep us happy. Cannabis can be used to mimic natural healthy hormones that eliminate stress and help restore balance.

Let's Talk About Getting High

How do drugs work? What happens when we use mood-altering substances? All chemicals in plants including coffee, cannabis, and chocolate mimic our hormones and substitute for naturally produced transmitters to activate different parts of our brain, gut, and heart. Cannabis mimics many, *many* different hormones that cause bliss and work to restore balance. It can help treat minor conditions and major disease. Getting high with cannabis means you're choosing to feel happy and relax.

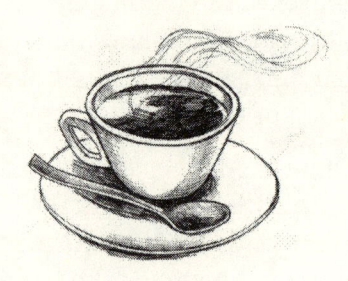

Psychoactive substances temporarily change the way our brain works to alter our perception, mood, consciousness, cognition, or behavior. Psychoactive substances in cannabis (THC) can be intoxicating or cause euphoria. Some people mistake euphoria as a negative side effect. Being happy has numerous therapeutic health benefits. One of the main reasons cannabis is life-saving for people with chronic illness or post-traumatic stress is because when you're happy it becomes possible to forget intense physical and mental pain, enjoy the present, laugh more, and relax. Getting high alters our perception of time, somehow slowing it down, to allow us to be more focused, present, and aware. When used in a trusted sacred space, it allows people to heal mentally and physically.

Cannabis works on receptors in the brain and body that cause a release of hormones to provide bliss and heighten our senses. We mentally become more present and aware. Cannabis does more than relax us—it helps our brain grow, develop, and protects the neurons in our entire body. It allows both sides of our brain to function and creates new pathways of learning. Receptors for cannabis and bliss hormones are everywhere. They are in every organ system, in nearly every cell, and are even inside of the tiny organelles within our cells. Cannabis changes our DNA to balances our hormones and provides us with more energy, relaxation, focus, and happiness.

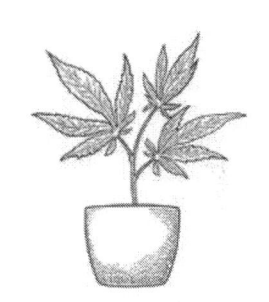

Using a drug that causes happiness and relaxation may not mean you feel that way at the beginning. It can take the right strain, dose, method, and environment. We all have different expectations and may not notice a change in behavior. Some people may need to use plant medicine regularly over a period of weeks in order to feel the full effect. Be warned not to get carried away when using cannabis at first. If you try *too* much at once, it can result in a lethargic, intense trip (which scares many people from wanting to try cannabis again).

Some people quickly find the right strain, dose, or method to feel happy and pain-free. For others it takes a little more trial and error. It is important to have faith that cannabis will help our body and mind heal, and to remember that cannabis is a tool not a cure-all.

Is there a line between medicinal, therapeutic, or recreational use? Getting *high* refers to entering a blissful state of physical and mental relaxation. Everyone experiences pain or emotional suffering and has times we feel low. Cannabis, and entheogens, can be used therapeutically to allow people with great suffering to experience happiness.

Mind & Body Interconnection

Most of us have a basic understanding of how our body works. We all know that there are systems in our body made of organs that are made of cells, but we may not fully understand how it's all connected. We know that we breathe air to fill our lungs with oxygen. That oxygen is transported through our blood to our brain to keep us alive. We all know that we eat and digest food to provide our brain and muscles with energy. So, there is a connection between our cells and different organs systems, but what is it? Why is it important?

Every cell in our body has receptors that communicate with one another. Our heart and gut are both a complex network of information, just like our brain, and have the ability to store information. Our three main networks work together to help us sense, feel, learn, and remember. Our brain, gut, and heart communicate by creating and transmitting chemical messages known as hormones. Hormones are released in high amounts during teenage years to help our body grow and mature, but more importantly they control our physical and mental health from birth to death. Hormones regulate our mood, appetite, heartbeat, memory, and pain sensation. Basically, these three organs communicate with hormones and work together to control how we think, feel, and act.

DID YOU KNOW YOU HAVE 3 BRAINS?

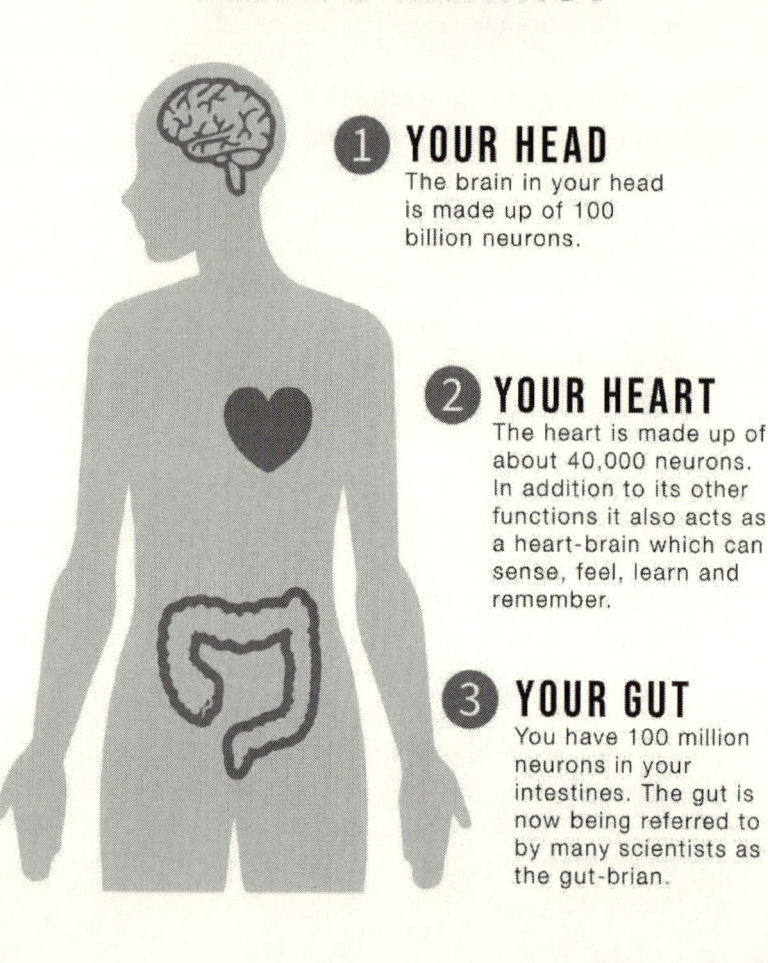

1 YOUR HEAD
The brain in your head is made up of 100 billion neurons.

2 YOUR HEART
The heart is made up of about 40,000 neurons. In addition to its other functions it also acts as a heart-brain which can sense, feel, learn and remember.

3 YOUR GUT
You have 100 million neurons in your intestines. The gut is now being referred to by many scientists as the gut-brian.

Our mental or emotional health is just as important as our physical health. Hormones are the source of our emotions and part of a massive interconnected communication system between our brain, heart, gut, and cells. Disease and illness are created from an imbalance in hormones—resulting in a dysfunction in the receptors that transmit chemical messages and control organ health. Hormones communicate between cells to start or stop organ function. When we are happy, we release bliss chemicals. When we are relaxed, we release healing hormones. When we are anxious or afraid, we release stress hormones. Our hormones are released in response to things we see, hear, touch, taste, smell, and think. Balancing all of our hormones is necessary in order to stay healthy mentally and physically. While it may not seem important that we create chemical messengers, an imbalance in our hormones is linked to every disease of the mind and body.

We essentially have two states of being for our body that are controlled by chemicals: alive or survive. When we are relaxed, the body releases beneficial chemicals so we can function properly, conserve energy, and heal. When we are afraid or stressed, we produce hormones that interrupt the ability to think, recover, and divert normal organ function in order to survive. We need to create beneficial chemicals and hormones through enjoyable activity and our diet to be healthy and feel alive.

Here are a few commonly known hormones or chemical messengers that we naturally produce:

<u>Bliss Chemicals</u>

- Dopamine (Reward)
- Opioid (Euphoria)
- Oxytocin (Love)
- Serotonin (Happy)
- Anandamide (Bliss)

<u>Beneficial Chemicals</u>

- GABA (Calm)
- Melatonin (Sleep)

<u>Stress Chemicals</u>

- Cortisol (Metabolism)
- Adrenaline (Panic)

Bliss hormones are released when we eat chocolate, drink coffee, stretch, get a massage, give or receive gifts, meditate, sing, dance, orgasm, breastfeed, exercise, and more. Bliss hormones motivate us to repeat similar activities and bond to others. Stress hormones are produced in times of fear. Fear and stress is something most of us avoid. Anger, sadness, humiliation, and a number of other emotions can make us feel uncomfortable. Trust your feelings and accept all emotions. Wisdom and healing comes from finding the courage to confront uncomfortable feelings. There is a tremendous breakthrough when you are not afraid of emotion and move past judgment.

Disease and illness happen when there is a prolonged imbalance in hormones. One of the most common imbalances is the lack of bliss hormones. We need to feel happy and relax daily to maintain good health. The importance of mental self-care is critical to creating bliss and our overall well-being. The importance of physical self-care through nutritious food, affectionate touch, stretching, exercise, laughing, intimate connection, and memorable experiences are critical to creating bliss hormones.

Food is the best source of medicine. Antioxidants, vitamins, minerals, healthy fat, complex carbohydrates, and plant protein give us energy and the ability to produce neurotransmitters and hormones. Many plants, herbs, and mushrooms contain anti-inflammatory and immune-boosting benefits that help our mind and body adapt to stress. Unfortunately many people go for something cheap and easy when hungry and eat processed food high in sugar and carbohydrates. Eating high amounts of simple carbohydrates daily puts your blood sugar and hormones on a roller-coaster causing certain organs to work over – time to maintain balance.

EXCESS CARBOHYDRATE CONSUMPTION
AFFECTS HEALTH, WEIGHT AND ENEGERY

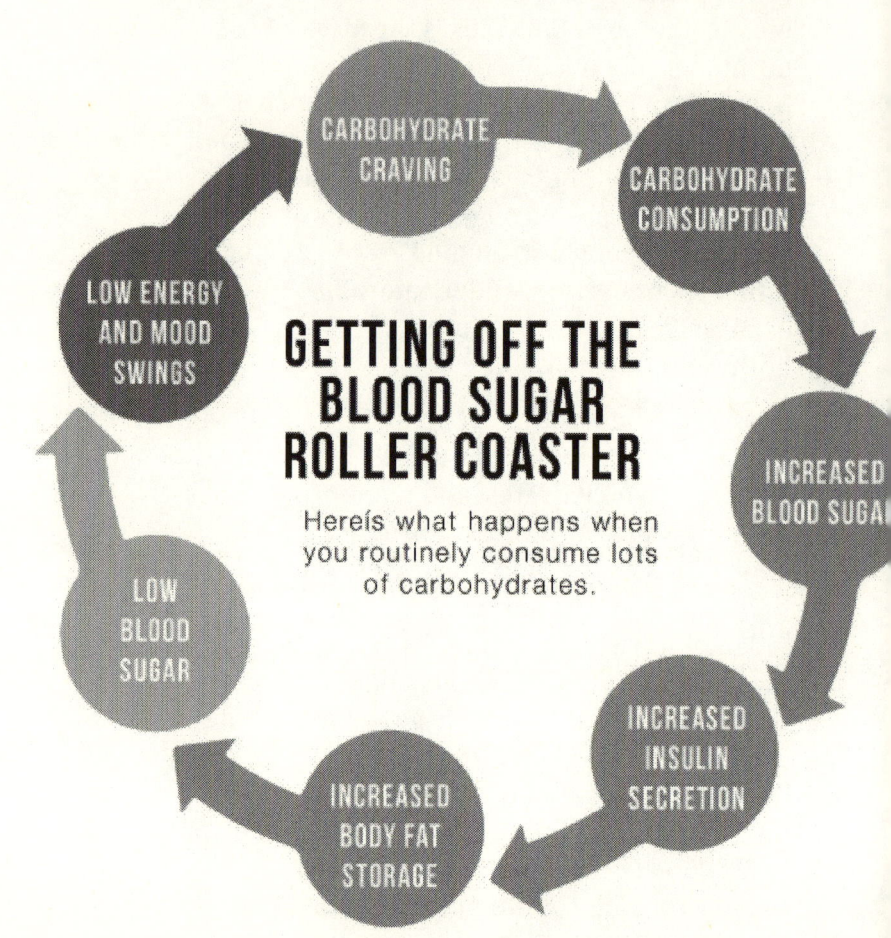

GETTING OFF THE BLOOD SUGAR ROLLER COASTER

Here's what happens when you routinely consume lots of carbohydrates.

- CARBOHYDRATE CRAVING
- CARBOHYDRATE CONSUMPTION
- INCREASED BLOOD SUGAR
- INCREASED INSULIN SECRETION
- INCREASED BODY FAT STORAGE
- LOW BLOOD SUGAR
- LOW ENERGY AND MOOD SWINGS

The second most common chemical imbalance is too much stress. Fear is healthy when it allows us to respond quickly and saves our lives in dangerous times. Repetitive stress, however, is toxic; causing a disruption in the communication process that prevents healing and promotes disease. Increased inflammation ages our body and mind causing our muscles, skin, bones, and brain to decay. Stress causes symptoms of chronic inflammation such as immune disorders, bone decay, cell death, gut issues, blood sugar issues, and an overall imbalance in our mind and body. Our entire body suffers when stress is prolonged.

We cannot be healthy if we are unhappy. We cannot heal if we do not relax. It's possible to overlook places where we carry physical and emotional pain if we do not bring awareness through practicing self-care. The root word of *wealth* means "health" or well-being. Most of us are programmed to believe working hard is necessary to be successful. Hard work means more money, quicker advancements in our career, and assumed greater overall satisfaction in life. The ideal lifestyle of material abundance, convenience, and ease is tempting. However, in the process of working hard, we can forget to relax and enjoy the moment. Having money provides us with basic needs, but wealth is truly measured by our level of happiness and overall health.

MIND
Difficulty concentrating, anxiety depression, irritability, mood

HEART
Increased cholesterol, Increased blood pressure, Risk of heart attack and stroke

JOINTS & MUSCLES
Increased inflammation, tension, aches and pains, muscle tightness, lower bone density

IMMUNE SYSTEM
Decreased immune function, lowered immune defenses, increased risk of becoming ill, increase in recovery time, Increased levels of inflammation

SKIN
Hair loss, dull/brittle hair, brittle nails, dry skin, acne, delayed tissue repair, psoriasis, eczema, rashes

GUT
Decreased nutrient absorption, reduced metabolism, ulcers, reflux, IBS, diabetes, nausea

REPRODUCTIVE SYSTEM
Decreased hormone production, decrease in libido, increase in PMS symptoms

IMPACT OF STRESS ON THE BODY

Dealing with Disease: Tools for Happiness

There are many ways to feel happy and get *high on life*. High, happy, and healthy all mean the same thing. Cannabis is just one of many tools that allows the body to relax and puts our mind at ease. It is only possible to be healthy if we are happy and take time to relax. Happiness isn't easy to attain, and relaxation can be hard to find if we don't have the tools necessary to build a foundation of healthy habits.

Healthy habits involve more than diet and exercise. Mental and emotional self-care is just as important as the physical aspect. Our emotions reflect the hormones being released in our body. We feel tired, anxious, or depressed when our hormones are off-balance. Being anxious or depressed weakens our immune system, and we become at risk for illness and infection. There are many tools and practices for building happiness that can be used to help our body relax and feel good in order to prevent disease or recover and heal.

Maintaining emotional and hormonal balance takes effort. While we may think that relaxation can be as simple as turning on the television, most forms of entertainment don't provide our mind with the rest it needs to unwind and heal.

Turning off electronics and distractions helps us tune into our body. Most of us choose to ignore minor aches and mild discomfort. Some even choose to ignore moderate pain or believe it's just part of getting *old*. It's better to bring attention and awareness to the places in our body where we feel hurt to provide ourselves with the love and care we need so we can get better and be well.

Powerful ancient tools and practices have been used for centuries in different cultures to allow our body and mind to reset. Yoga and massage can help bring awareness and heal the places in our body where we carry physical pain. Meditation and talk therapy can help us find and heal the places in our mind where we feel pain and fear. Love and gratitude help to heal a wounded spirit and inspire us with hope. Plant medicine allows us to feel happy, relaxed, and balanced. Positive thinking gives us the courage to create happiness for ourselves. Food is a great source of medicine and plays an important role in maintaining emotional balance.

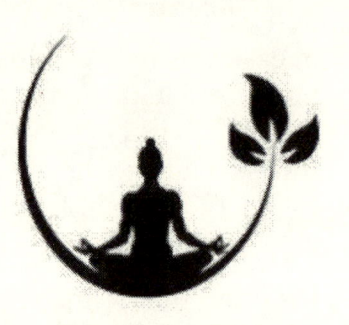

Healthy habits may not seem that important, but it is the only way to maintain happiness. Men are not encouraged to prioritize mental or emotional self-care practices but rather be tough and reserved. Unfortunately, things like yoga and meditation are seen by many as a feminine practice. Expressing yourself emotionally can be seen as dramatic and unnecessary. Getting a massage can be seen as pampering. However, when we practice self-care, our body begins to crave the attention it needs. People who stretch or get a massage often are mindfully connected with their body and become aware of tension in their muscles. A person in-tune with their body can feel when something is out of balance in their muscles or joints and take care of the issue before it becomes a problem. It is much better to treat the problem and nip issues in the bud rather than to ignore pain (or uncomfortable emotions).

Cannabis can be used to enhance mind-body awareness during meditation, yoga, exercise, and day-to-day activities. The perception and awareness of the position and movement of our body can be a hard sense to develop. Many people feel uncomfortable in their skin and focus on their imperfections. It can be hard to get in tune with our body when we reject how we look and feel flawed, fat, or weak. Meditation can be hard for people with unsettled thoughts or emotions. For some people just the idea of yoga or massage makes them feel uncomfortable. Low self-esteem, anxiety, or discomfort prevents people from fully participating and enjoying healthy activities. Cannabis allows us to eliminate uncomfortable thoughts and focus on our muscle movement. It also helps to decrease inflammation and help post-workout recovery.

Our perception shapes how we interpret life experiences and release hormones. Many of us get jobs to pay bills and are forced to budget or save whatever we have. A lot of people create careers out of jobs that have little meaning other than income or title. Feeling forced to work in a position or job that doesn't bring us joy depletes happy hormones and makes us feel worthless. Relationships that don't bring us joy make us isolated. Responsibilities that become obligations make us feel burdened. When we start to become disconnected from life, it slowly sucks the joy out of what we do and makes us feel depleted and empty at the end of our day. When we settle for being content with what *is* rather than seeking to be happy, we forget what it's like to have joy inspire our mind and body.

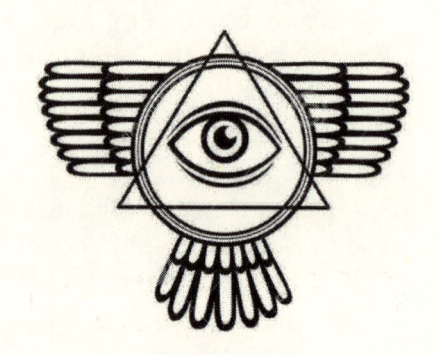

There are many ways to feel happy, and there are different levels of happiness. Some forms of happiness are fleeting. Healthy habits deepen our ability to connect with ourselves, connect with others, and increase our happiness. Wise people realize that success follows happiness—not the other way around. If you spend all your time trying to be successful, then you may never find happiness.

Put faith in love rather than luck or random chance. Believe healing is possible. The opportunities we have for happiness can only be seen when we have an open heart and positive attitude. Connection is the cure to unhappiness. The more interconnected we are to life, the more often we feel happy and healthy. When we care about our jobs, partners, family, and duties, it deeply fills us with a continual sense of value, appreciation, pride, and joy. It becomes easier to feel inspired and motivated, rather than obligated and resentful. We appreciate the things in our lives, rather than feel envious of what we don't have.

Many people are programmed to live life according to family and society expectations rather than their own authentic aspirations. Certain emotions or desires are taboo and become repressed and avoided. Prejudice and phobias limit people from connecting to their authentic emotions, desires, and happiness. Emotions aren't innately good or bad. All emotions can be expressed and processed in a way that is healthy or unhealthy. Fear can guide us to safety. Fear can also trick us into living a boring life. Confidence and compassion allow us to surrender control and make changes to grow happiness. Having a positive attitude and taking responsibility changes the way we respond and react to situations. We can evolve rather than repeat mistakes.

When we are not labeling ourselves or others for how we look or act, it becomes easy to notice that humans are programmed by their environment by nature. Our brain develops pathways based on our actions and creates habitual patterns that teach our body what to expect, avoid, and crave.

Far too many children grow up in an unhealthy environment and develop negative coping mechanisms that help them survive. Neglect, abuse, and impoverishment wreak havoc on a child's wellness. Many survivors typically find drugs allow them to feel happy and at peace by replacing the natural chemicals they are lacking. It also gives a sense of control, as they may have learned few tools that create happiness. Victims of abuse can disassociate from their emotions to the point where they feel nothing is wrong. The process of reprogramming the brain can take months, years, or decades. It takes time to build trust and develop healthy habits.

Children in dysfunctional families create negative coping mechanisms in order to survive. A child can also take on the negative coping mechanisms of their parents, or develop them in order to be accepted by their peers. As adults, many of us search for ways to escape stress and rely on the negative coping mechanisms we developed while young. We can escape reality through becoming obsessed with nearly any substance or activity: reading, eating, working, watching television, using social media, sex, religious practices, socializing,, pharmaceuticals, alcohol, caffeine, nicotine, and other drugs. The chemicals in plants that help us feel happy or high are innately good. In fact, most people get addicted to a substance providing a chemical that their body isn't naturally producing in order to help them maintain balance (and control). However, just like anything else cannabis can be abused when used solely to escape reality. No substance or activity should be used to fill an emotional void. Negative coping mechanisms can be created out of boredom, or as a survival tactic. People who use cannabis and entheogens are stigmatized, labeled as *drug addicts* or *stoners*, and shunned. Chemicals in pharmaceuticals, alcohol, or coffee carry fewer stigmas even though they have a high risk of abuse, addiction, and physical dependency. Any chemical can be used therapeutically for well-being, or abused to escape reality and maintain trapped in fantasy. Our time is best spent doing enjoyable activities that inspire our creativity and leave us with a sense of accomplishment, gratitude, and peace.

The majority of us can use help reprogramming our brain to eliminate negative coping mechanisms. Our perspective is limited, and mind-altering medicines allow us to transcend our hardwiring or mental and physical conditioning. Cannabis is one of the best tools to retrain your brain. It can help you see the bigger picture. The feeling that something is wrong in our life, mind, or body is detrimental to our health. Cannabis can do more than help us forget our worries—it helps you forget that there is anything *wrong* with you. It takes courage and a positive mindset to make the changes necessary to be healthy. Mind-altering plants allow us to heal mental wounds and shift our perspective, so we can see the bigger picture and inspire change.

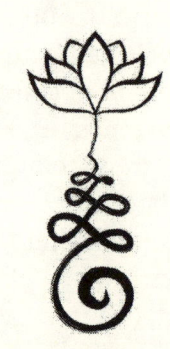

Many people are faced with *chronic* or *incurable* diseases because they were unable to recognize or treat the initial issue. We expect that only doctors are qualified and able to deal with disease. When we put blind faith in health professionals, it becomes easy to forget that *you* are the most important member of the healing team. Remember that it is possible to get better and be well through routine self-care combined with the belief that healing is possible. A negative mind-set and suppressing emotions reduce the ability to heal.

We heal from disease or trauma by connecting with our emotions and taking care of our body. It is possible to restore physical and mental balance with dedicated self-care. A healthy diet, restful sleep, deep breathing, meditation, affectionate touch, relaxation, positive thinking, stretching, and enjoyable exercise provide us with energy necessary to deal with stressful moments. Plant medicine allows us to replace any missing hormones and overcome disease.

Keep in mind that the more serious the disease, the more commitment it takes to restore balance. Using cannabis daily for a period of months or years does not mean you will become addicted for life. Plant medicine is not a cure-all on its own for medical conditions, but frees patients controlled by disease. Cannabis allows users to improve their quality of life by managing symptoms of stress and illness. Positive lifestyle changes and multiple therapies help healing occur and reduce dependency on medication. Multiple tools should be used to maintain balance. Diet, massage, music, meditation, and enjoyable exercise are just a few examples of ways to enhance our endocannabinoid system naturally, increase effectiveness of plant medicine, decrease dependency and cravings, and restore balance.

For people trapped in victimizing or self-harming behavior, chasing the high and release of bliss chemicals can become burdensome. The amount of time and resources it can take continue to chase the high can become burdensome. There is a line between use and abuse. We all must work to enjoy life in various ways, develop deep connections, and use chemical substances with care. The longer we continue to avoid making the changes necessary to deal with stress or pain, the more systemic disease becomes. It is possible to intervene when trapped in a viscous cycle. We can re-parent our inner child to heal the wounds of neglect, abuse, or impoverishment with the help of therapeutic tools. When our jobs and relationships lack meaning we feel empty, and we seek sanctuary through external comforts. Unresolved emotional stress and negative thought patterns can lead to self-satisfying and co-dependent tendencies. Instead, triumph over pain and fear with love and understanding by creating an inner sanctuary of bliss.

The first part of the recovery process means believing that healing physical pain and psychological trauma *is possible*. That allows a person to shift their perspective, prioritize self-care, embrace the natural world and consider cannabis as a bridge to recovery. When we settle our mind and let go of anxious thoughts, it gives our inner voice a chance to guide us with wisdom. Internalizing negative criticisms causes unnecessary stress and prevents us from making authentic decisions. Recovery takes place when we prioritize self-care and lead a happy authentic life. Harmony is built on a foundation of positive thinking and self-care.

Tools for Self-Care

Mental:

- Be Authentic & Genuine
- Positive Attitude
- Meditation
- Therapy
- Deep Breathing
- Support & Encouragement
- Adaptogens/Herbs/Plant Medicine, THC

Physical:

- Massage & Stretching
- Strength Training
- Nourishing Food
- Intimacy
- Restful Sleep
- Antioxidants, Anti-inflammatories, Probiotics
- Cannabis/Herbs/Plant medicine, CBD

Spiritual:

- Awareness
- Compassion
- Entheogens
- Forgiveness
- Gratitude
- Generosity

The Endocannabinoid System

The endocannabinoid system (**ECS**) is the most widespread receptor system in the human body. Endocannabinoids are naturally occurring transmitters that we produce in our brain and body. From initiating uterine attachment during conception through releasing growth hormones in adolescence—it plays the most important role in sustaining health and well-being.

The ECS functions to help us relax, eat, sleep, and forget painful memories. It regulates both our mind and body including fertility, mood, appetite, pain sensation, memory, development of neurons, bone regeneration, and learning ability. It restores a state of balance, or homeostasis, in the immune system, reduces pain, and helps us relax and experience bliss. Due to the stigmatization of cannabis, it's no wonder why most people have never heard about the endocannabinoid system. Discovered in 1988, many doctors and health professionals are still unaware we even have one. It's unfortunate that many people are unaware that we have a natural system that restores harmony and allows us to heal. Disease occurs when it stops working correctly. ECS dysfunction is linked to every chronic medical condition.

Cannabinoids are the key to healthy living. Happiness and harmony are created when cannabinoids enter our bloodstream. Cannabinoids regulate our mind, heart, gut, and entire body and balance our hormones. Cannabinoids are naturally created in our bodies and in cannabis plants. Endocannabinoids are naturally produced by our body during exercise, meditation, laughter, deep breathing, and singing. Endocannabinoids are also called endorphins. Plant-based cannabinoids fit into hormone receptors and activate them. Phytocannabinoids or plant-based cannabinoids can be found in cannabis, black pepper, cacao, Japanese liverwort, echinacea, black truffles, kava, electric daisy, and other plants. Plant cannabinoids mimic our natural transmitters and hormones.

Stress causes our body to go into fight, flight, or freeze response and disrupts the natural balance. Toxins, free-radicals, and detrimental proteins are released in response to stress and speed up inflammation, aging and death. Cannabinoids are created and released to stimulate the relaxation response so we can heal, recover, restore and learn. People suffering with disease have a cannabinoid deficiency. Cannabinoids are proven to help protect our neurons, enhance brain function, and form new pathways.

ECS receptors are wide-spread and overlap with many other chemical receptor systems. Anandamide is the name of a chemical we naturally create and commonly referred to as the "bliss" hormone. It inhibits adrenaline, helping provide relaxation. **THC** is the cannabinoid in cannabis that activates receptors in the system to provide euphoria and relaxation and mimics our naturally occurring bliss hormone, anandamide. It provides pain relief, joy, sleep, and healthy appetite. **CBD** is another cannabinoid in cannabis that works indirectly on receptors in order to prevent the breakdown of bliss hormones. Cannabis is medicinal because of the many actions it has on various chemical receptor systems. Cannabinoids interact with many other systems, helping to regulate pain, appetite, mood, cancer, inflammation, blood pressure, blood sugar, metabolism, and the immune system. It's amazing how many benefits cannabis can have on our health and well-being.

Cannabinoid (CB) receptors regulate many important transmitter pathways in the human body. They control the flow of signals that are being sent between cells. It stabilizes our brain, bones, organs and immune system by allowing us to relax, heal, and experience joy.

CB receptors are created naturally inside cells and move to the membrane where they wait ready to be activated by endocannabinoids.

CB1 receptors are mainly in the brain and nervous system. THC and anandamide activate CB1 receptors causing euphoria that relieves depression, nausea, and pain. Many neurological and mental problems are associated with CB1 receptor dysfunction. THC increases blood flow and opens the airway, but it does not control heart rate or breath—making it impossible to overdose. There are no receptors found in the medulla or brainstem. CB1 receptors can be found in the brain, nervous system, thyroid, airway, liver, adrenals, uterus, prostate, testes, eye, stomach, pancreas, heart, bones, and digestive tract.

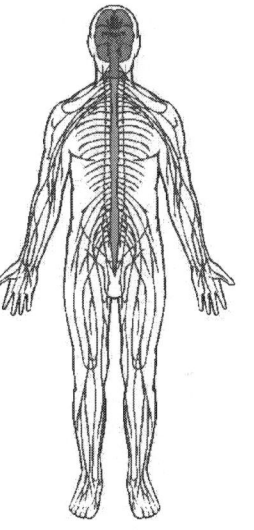

CB2 receptors are in the immune system and peripheral organs. Many medicinal properties of THC, and beta-caryophyllene, are attributed to activating CB2 receptors. Autoimmune disorders, chronic inflammation, Alzheimer's, and Chron's are associated with CB2 receptor dysfunction. CB2 receptors are found in the eye, stomach, heart, pancreas, bones, digestive tract, and skin. Cannabinoids that activate CB2 receptors increase anti-inflammatory response, neuroprotection and bone development. They also modulate dopamine activity, making it a potent treatment for addiction.

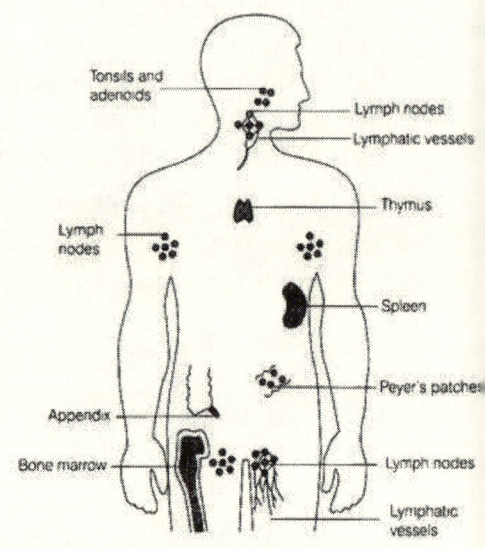

Cannabis affects other receptors besides CB1 and CB2. It interacts with nearly every other receptor system including serotonin, dopamine, oxytocin, opioid, melatonin, and GABA. THC fits into our cannabinoid, serotonin, dopamine, and opioid receptors and activates the production and release of hormones. CBD fits into our cannabinoid, serotonin, and dopamine receptors to prevent the breakdown of hormones (but is not able to activate the receptors on its own). Pets and Children have endocannabinoid systems that can benefit from cannabis use. Many parents and pet owners are reluctant to use medical cannabis due to the lack of support by health providers and their community.

Cannabinoids cause nearly every cell to produce bliss hormones. When we rub cannabis lotion on or get a massage, we release hormones to make our skin happy. When we smoke cannabis or meditate, we make our brain happy. When we eat cannabis or a healthy meal, we make our digestive system happy. Chemotherapy patients find relief from pain and nausea when using cannabis and alternative medicine. Opioid patients find a reduction in the amount of medication necessary to relieve symptoms while decreasing their tolerance, reducing side-effects, and eliminating withdrawal. People suffering from chronic depression or anxiety find the ability to be happy and peaceful. Children with seizures, Tourette's, and ADHD find relief without becoming a pharma-zombie. Cannabis shows a therapeutic potential for all diseases affecting humans.[1]

---

[1] Pal Pacher, George Kunos, "Modulating the eCB system in health and disease: successes and failures," (2013)

Marijuana: Paranoia & Propaganda

It's important to talk about the power of thought. Our mind can be the most powerful healing tool when given the chance. It can also prevent us from surrendering control or allowing ourselves to enjoy being happy. When approaching cannabis use, everyone has a different level of comfort with the idea of getting high. Many people are worried about being noticeably high. The fear of being too happy or high is due to decades of stigma. If you believe that getting high will make you lazy, clumsy, addicted, or forgetful, then it becomes easy to blame cannabis and become lazy, clumsy, and forgetful. If you are worried about how cannabis may alter your state of mind, or how others may judge you, then it becomes easy to become paranoid when using certain forms of cannabis. Many people with severe disease or illness witness that cannabis has the power to help them heal and allow them lead a successful productive life. Believing cannabis is a positive influence makes it easier to use it as a tool for happiness.

Whether or not your family is accepting of cannabis use, it can be hard to be accepted by everyone all the time. Our thoughts and preconceived ideas alter our awareness and decision-making process. The opinion of others can heavily influence our perception and can alter how we react to drugs, especially at first. Feeling uncomfortable with cannabis might make it hard to experience or notice the effects. If someone believes that getting high is bad for them, then letting go mentally in order to fully experience the effects can be difficult. Instead of enjoying the heightened state of being, it can be unnerving. Cannabis should be used in a safe space where you can be comfortable and relaxed. We need to provide a physical and mental space to allow cannabis to work effectively. Scientific research has discovered beneficial chemicals in cannabis help stabilize our flow of hormones. Faith that cannabis will help healing take place makes it more effective as medicine. Cannabis is much more beneficial when used in a relaxed setting without fear of judgment.

Some people will try the wrong strain, dose, or method and give up before seeing results. Others get scared after trying too much. For some, the taboo is too much to even want to try cannabis at all. At first, it can be hard to relax with the idea of using cannabis. Cannabis is still heavily stigmatized, and many people are nervous when walking into a cannabis store for the first time. We all have at least one friend or family member that thinks smoking or using weed is *bad* or for *stoners*. Cannabis was used as medicine for centuries and highly regarded for its many medicinal uses. In the early 1900s cannabis was rebranded as *marijuana*. Harry Anslinger headed the commission that spearheaded the campaign to help spread propaganda that demonized cannabis in news and films and made marijuana illegal. Movies such as *Tell Your Children* (also known as *Reefer Madness,* released in 1936) convinced audiences that if you tried cannabis, even once, it would lead to uncontrollable urges like premarital sex, murder, and insanity.

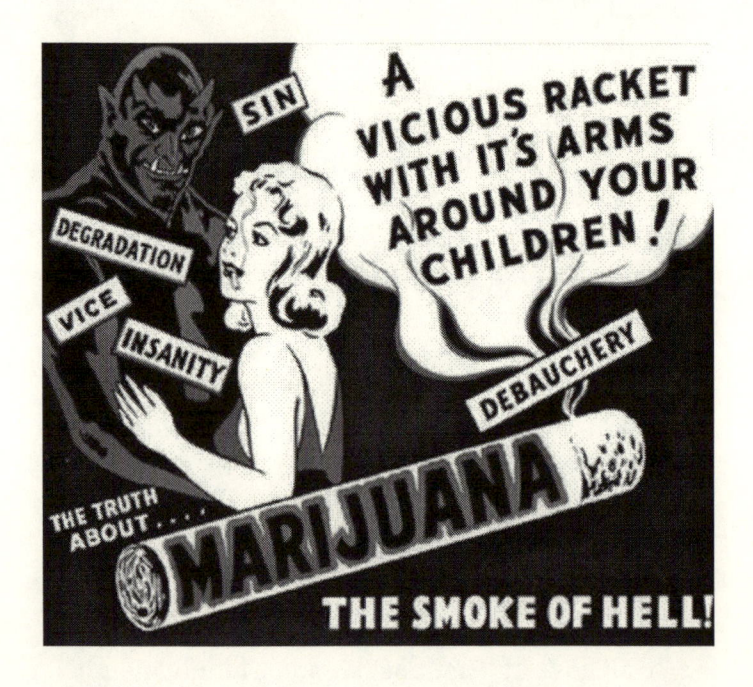

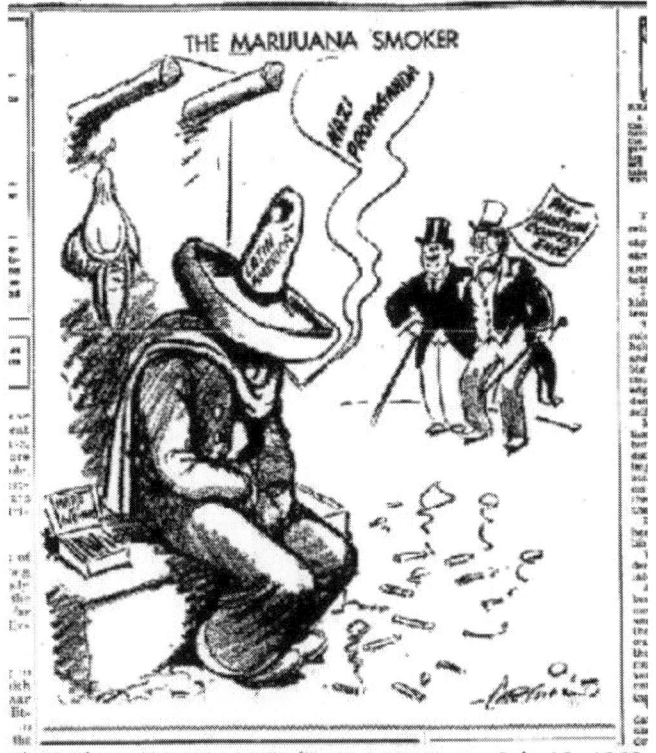

The Vidette Messenger, Indiana newspaper - July 19, 1940

The fear that Mexican and Black men would tempt white girls fueled racist and ignorant opinions. Even though it was proven through research that cannabis was in fact non-addictive, non-toxic, and a potential cure to many diseases, research was brushed off and buried for about a century. Some newspapers cited marijuana as the reason behind violent crimes.

THE OGDEN STANDARD

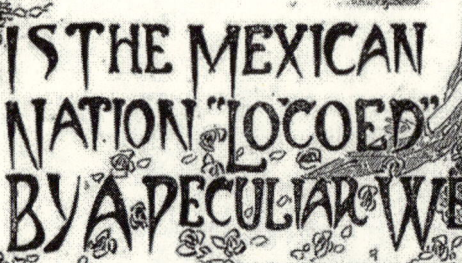

MAGAZINE SECTION — OGDEN, UTAH, SATURDAY, SEPTEMBER 25, 1915 — MAGAZINE SECTION

IS THE MEXICAN NATION "LOCOED" BY A PECULIAR WEED?

Deadly Marihuana Rolled In Cigarettes, Becomes the Curse Of the Southern Republic and May Account For the "Bravery" Of "Greaser" Bandits Who Defy the United States—The Insanity Of Queen Carlotta Is Accounted For In the Familiar Historical Legend Of the Poisoned Tea

GENERAL VENUSTIANO CARRANZA

GENERAL PANCHO VILLA

CARLOTTA, EMPRESS OF MEXICO

MAXIMILIAN, EMPEROR OF MEXICO

Nixon and Regan reinforced the stigmatization of cannabis—launching the War on Drugs and "Just Say No" campaign that allowed for the continued imprisonment of people of color. It's wrong that cannabis was viewed as negative or harmful. The only harm that comes from cannabis is the possibility of getting arrested for using or selling it. The idea that we can be happy by living a relaxed lifestyle where we are connected to nature or mindfully present is associated with *hippies*. We have been misguided for decades under perpetual xenophobia lead by racist politicians, for-profit prisons, and pharmaceutical companies.

It's bizarre that a natural substance that can treat so many medical conditions, with little side-effects or no risk of overdose is less acceptable than other "drugs." Many prescription pills would no longer be used if cannabis became publicly available. Forbes published an article in April 2018 citing numerous recent studies that show legal states have lower opioid use and about 25% less overdose. Two months earlier, Forbes published an article on a New York Senator Kirstin Gillibrand calling out Big Pharma on opposing cannabis legalization. The article noted that in 2016, a major manufacturer of fentanyl, synthetic THC, and opioid products, Insys Therapeutics, donated $500,000 to help defeat cannabis legalization in Arizona. The truth is many pharmaceutical companies lobby for the prohibition of cannabis. Pharmaceutical medicines replicate chemicals in plants or are derived from them. While cannabis and other natural plant medicines have been stigmatized and prohibited in America and many other countries, we continue to manufacture synthetic drugs based on illegal substances that provide more harm than benefit. The acceptance of pharmaceutical medicine meant that many people over the past century turned away from natural medicine. Unfortunately, it's led to an over-prescription of anti-depressants and pain killers. Since 1999, the number of annual deaths in American due to opioid overdose has grown from roughly 17,000 to 70,000. Cannabis is helping put an end to the opioid epidemic.

The United States Department of Health and Human Services patented cannabis as an antioxidant and neuroprotectant in 2003 while the government simultaneously imprisoned people for its use. Federal classification of cannabis as a Schedule 1 Substance has blocked access to cannabis and entheogenic medicines that could benefit millions of people with grave conditions. Cannabis use is heavily stigmatized and criminalized. As the *Refer Madness* era begins to come to an end, there are still many people unaware of the medical benefits of cannabis or how to approach cannabis use. Doctors, health care professionals, and the public are poorly informed about the endocannabinoid system. Contemporary medicine tends to separate the organs in our body into mutually exclusive functions. It is unwise to do so as our mind, body, emotions, and environment have an influence and impact on our health. Cannabis is one of many health tools that should be combined with other therapies and used in a relaxed environment.

Chronic pain and illness motivate people to seek relief. Many who are faced with disease and are unable to participate in life suffer similar symptoms (pain, insomnia, anxiety, depression) that cause the disease to worsen. Once you start to experience the symptoms of a disease, it becomes impossible to treat without serious self-care. It takes more than a pill or a joint to heal. Cannabis treats major disease and alleviates suffering. When combined with other forms of therapy, cannabis can help with the symptoms of nearly every medical condition. Cannabis can help end the opioid epidemic, replace alcohol and detrimental drugs, and eliminate the need for pharmaceuticals. Cannabis is an exit drug and a gateway to enlightenment.

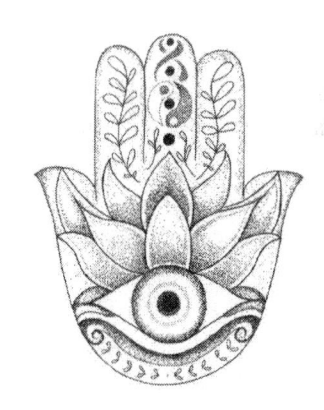

Cannabis Plant

Cannabis is an annual plant (it completes its life cycle in one year). Plants are either male or female. Female plants produce flowers that contain sticky trichomes (glandular hairs) with cannabinoids and terpenes (scent chemicals). These sticky little trichomes are what give cannabis plants medicinal value. Cannabis flowers are overflowing with scent and flavor. The plant is related to the rose family, which also contains strawberries, peaches, apples, almonds, pears, and figs, among others. Some strains or varieties of cannabis have a pungent, skunky aroma while others have a sweet citrus or floral small. The scent chemicals play an important role in the medicinal value.

Terpenes and cannabinoids develop differently depending on many factors. Strain is only part of the equation when determining effect. Growing conditions, light exposure, part of the plant, and harvest time affect the development of the plant and resulting effect. The chemical makeup of the same strain of cannabis varies depending on the quality of soil, age of plant, and part of plant. The same strain usually has similar effects, but not always, as there are minor differences in genetics, growing season, harvesting time, and the extraction or infusion process. Plants grown outdoors are exposed to the entire light

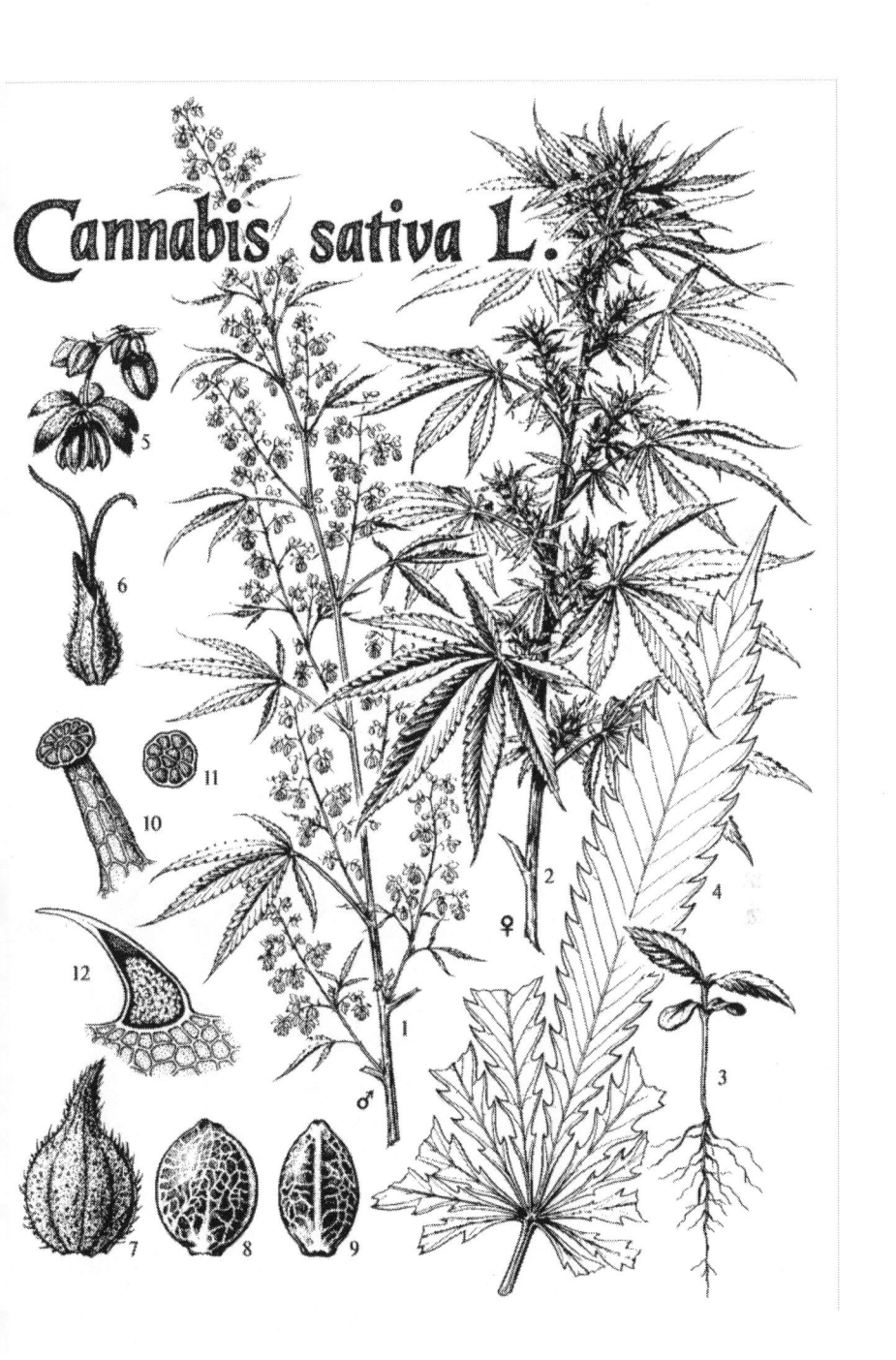

Cannabis sativa L.

spectrum and produce the best medicine when grown with care in fertile organic soil. Outdoor grows are much better for the environment.

Cannabis is a hyperaccumulator and bioregulator, meaning it absorbs chemicals, heavy metals, radiation and toxins from the air, soil, and water. Cannabis plants can easily contain toxins if grown in an unhealthy environment. Organic farming is necessary to ensure cannabis medicine is safe for consumption.

The generalizing of cannabis strains into Sativa, Indica, and Hybrid is a helpful basic tool for new users. But it is only a steppingstone to learning more about terpenes and cannabinoids. Cannabis effects come down to the terpenes (pungency) and cannabinoids (potency). *Cannabis sativa* and *Cannabis indica* were named based on their size and leaf pattern (and not effects, cannabinoids, or DNA). *Sativa* plants grow taller with their flowers spaced further apart and have narrow leaves. *Indica* plants are shorter plants with broad leaves. "Sativa" strains are generally more uplifting and energetic, while "Indica" strains are generally better for relaxation and sleep. However, generalizing effects into such broad categories isn't necessarily accurate.

Hemp

Hemp CBD products are available at most grocery stores now. Unlike cannabis products, hemp isn't tested for heavy metals, pesticides, and contaminants the same way as cannabis products. Hemp is dramatically less effective for serious medical conditions, being entirely *in*effective in most cases. Hemp-based CBD products can be help treat mild conditions in some cases, but hemp products have CBD alone and they do not enough THC or terpenes to stimulate the entourage effect. While CBD can help keep you happy if you already have a healthy, functioning system, THC is necessary to make us feel happy and treat pain or serious illness.

Hemp-based CBD products are helping to de-stigmatize cannabis and can carry a great placebo effect. Hemp or distilled cannabis products are useful for users suffering from minor pain or mild anxiety. If hemp-based products work for you, then cannabis products are likely to be even more effective. If hemp products aren't working that well—then try whole plant cannabis products. Keep in mind that most companies are trying to profit off people rather than help them get better. Hemp companies are making money on the misconception that cannabis and hemp products have similar effects—they do not.

"Hemp" is a term used to classify fibrous cannabis varieties having a minute amount of THC (below 0.3%) and small amounts of CBD. Hemp, Mary Jane, weed, ganja, mota, bud, and reefer are just names for the same plant. During the 1930s, the government legally separated "marijuana" from "hemp." Technically speaking, there are five chemotaxonomic varieties or types of cannabis. That means plants can be separated based on their chemical makeup rather than plant size and leaf pattern. *Hemp* plants are fibrous varieties and produce fewer resin flowers with less terpenes. CBD is a byproduct of hemp plants, and has a far less medicinal value than cannabis plants. Hemp plants are best used for their oil and fiber.

Entourage Effect & Whole Plant Medicine

Whole plant medicine uses the *entire* plant instead of isolated components. That means using the flowers, leaves, stems, and roots. The most beneficially healing experience comes from consuming whole plant medicine.

The entourage effect is what makes whole plant cannabis medicine so valuable. Cannabinoids are enhanced by scent chemicals[2]. Cannabis potency (percentage/milligrams of THC/CBD) only accounts for part of the effect. Sedation, stimulation, euphoria, and other effects from different varieties of cannabis come from the fragrance or scent chemicals called terpenes. There are over four hundred chemicals in whole cannabis plant medicine. The entourage effect comes from complex interactions between chemicals. Cannabis contains more than 140 cannabinoids, 200 terpenes, and 20 flavonoids. Terpenes provide scent and flavonoids flavor. They play an important role in the survival of the plant by attracting pollinators and detouring predators. Terpenes interact with cannabinoids to enhance and balance the experience. Certain

---

[2] Russo, Ethan B. "Taming THC: potential cannabis synergy and phytocannabinoid-terpenoid entourage effects" *British journal of pharmacology* vol. 163,7 (2011): 1344-64.

chemicals work with each other as synergists while others counteract each other. CBD and THC work together to reduce pain and inflammation while counteracting anxiety. Certain terpenes allow cannabinoids to travel more effectively through our system and provide a more intense effect. It's not as simple as 1 + 1 = 2. The chemicals in cannabis combine in complex ways.

A standardized cannabis extract goes through the process of being distilled, refined, or isolated to guarantee the amount of a specific medicinal component. The intent of standardization is to provide consistency from batch-to-batch during manufacturing. That means when you go in to buy a cannabis product, it will have the same amount of medicine each time. If a cannabis consumer is focusing more on the number of milligrams THC or CBD in each product, they lose sight of the importance of all the other hundreds of chemicals. Nature did not intend for standardization and mass production.

Synthetic or pharmaceutical medicine is produced artificially in a lab based on a single chemical structure. The benefits of cannabis cannot be simplified from 700 chemicals into one. When concentrating one chemical at the expense of others, it unintentionally eliminates or neglects components that contribute to the entourage effect. CBD and THC alone have little to no therapeutic use. Distillates and hemp products carry a fraction of the chemicals in cannabis. Most products in legalized states are made from distillate. Standardized and synthetic medicine is less effective and harder to dose than whole plant medicine. It's like going from a first-aid kit to a band-aid.

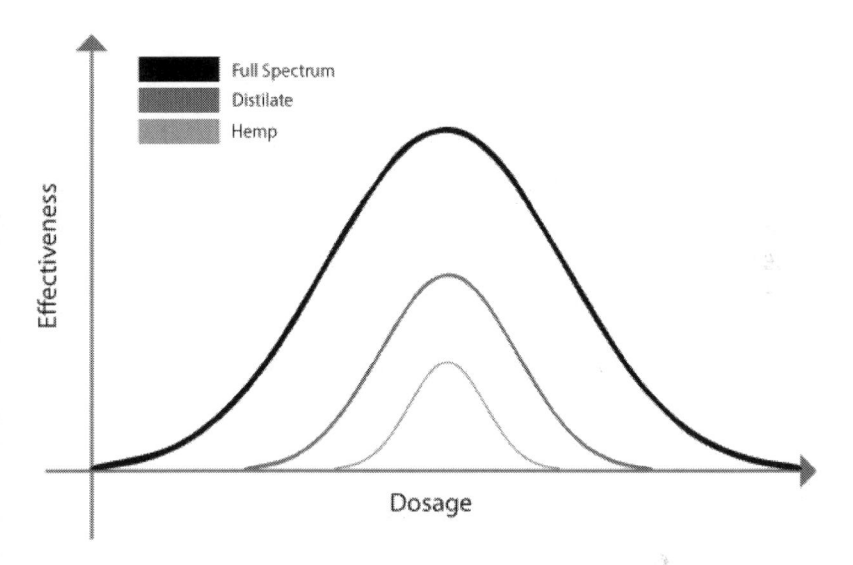

Legend: Full Spectrum, Distilate, Hemp

Y-axis: Effectiveness; X-axis: Dosage

Full Spectrum CBD vs Distilate vs Hemp

Children with seizures have reported the necessity of terpenes and THC in trace amounts when taking CBD medication. With over four hundred different chemicals in the cannabis plant, it is important for anyone with serious disease to use whole plant medicine. Distillates, isolates, hemp, and synthesized pharmaceutical medicine is typically limited in the scope of treatment and often comes with side-effects.

Limited molecules do not exhibit the entourage effect and have a smaller dosing curve, meaning it's harder to dose and less effective. Whole plant cannabis products can be made at home.

It is possible to determine which products are made with distillate when purchasing in a store. Certain products will say "full plant spectrum" as a marketing gimmick. They can be distillated oils with a limited number of cannabis or terpenes reintroduced (which is not the same quality as whole plant medicine). The term "full-specturm" refers to whole plant medicine, but is not regulated with cannabis product labeling. An easy way to tell by-eye is to examine the color of your oil, tincture, capsule, or vape cartridge. Distilled oil stripped of many cannabinoids and terpenes are typically gold or straw in color. Products that are green or amber contain a full-spectrum profile. Chocolates and other edibles that have little or no cannabis flavor are made with distillate.

When trying cannabis, users are also encouraged to experiment with different strains, ratios, and cannabinoids. THC and CBD interact with different cannabinoid receptors and areas of the body. When used together, patients find peak medicinal effectiveness by activating multiple receptors, preventing cannabinoid breakdown, and stimulating both sides of the brain. THC and CBD together create harmony so our mind and body can heal.

Ratio (CBD:THC)	Effects
0:1 THC Only	Intoxicating, Euphoria, Side-effects for novices
1:2	Uplifted emotions with calmer thoughts. Mild side-effects, Intense Pain Relief, Sleep Aid
1:1	Greatest therapeutic benefits: Moderate Pain relief, Anti-inflammatory, Neuroprotectant, Bone Growth, Balance Gut, Tranquil
2:1	Mild sedation and relaxation. Anti-psychotic, anti-inflammatory, Mild pain relief, Weak euphoria
20:1 CBD-Rich	Reduce anxiety, inflammation, seizures
Hemp CBD Only	Mild anti-inflammatory, mind-anti-psychotic, possibly no effect

Common Plant Cannabinoids

The following is an abreviated list of phytocannabinoids found in cannabis. There are over 120 plant cannabinoids discovered so far.

CBGA is the precursor to CBG, THCA, CBDA, and CBCA. Cannabis plants harvested early will have higher amounts of CBGA. Medicinal benefits include anti-inflammation.

CBG can be used for pain releif, inflammation, bacterial or fungal infection, bone growth, and inhibition of cell growth in certain cancer.

THCA is the precursor to delta-9 THC. It is found in raw cannabis. Medicinal benefits include anti-inflammatory, neuroprotective, anti-epileptic, and the inhibition of cell growth in tumors and certain cancer. THCA is far less psychoactive than THC and provides many similar benefits.

THCV is found in heated or aged cannabis. Medicinal benefits include suppressing the appetite, reducing seizures, reducing blood sugar levels, and stimulating bone growth.

THC or delta-9 THC occurs when THCA is heated or aged. It is the psychoactive component of cannabis. Medicinal benefits include acute pain relief, appetite stimulation, reduction of vomiting and nausea, and suppression of muscle spasms.

CBN is the final stage of THC and is found in aged flower. Health effects of CBN include pain relief, reduction of muscle spasms, and anti-insomnia.

CBDA is the precursor to CBD and found in certain varieties of raw cannabis. Health benefits include anti-inflammatory and inhibition of tumor growth in certain cancer.

CBDV is found in heated or aged cannabis. Research has recently discovered it as a powerful anti-epileptic.

CBD is produced when CBDA is heated or aged. Medicinal benefits include pain relief, anti-inflammation, appetite stimulant, reduction of nausea and contractions in the small intestine, anxiety and depression relief, seizure reduction, suppression of muscle spasms, blood sugar regulation, anti-bacterial, promotion of bone growth, and inhibition of cell growth in tumors. People suffering from arthritis, MS, neuropathy pain, and neurodegeneration are encouraged to use CBD-rich medicine daily.

CBCA is the precursor to CBC and is found in raw cannabis. Medicinal uses include treatment for fungal infection and bacterial growth.

CBC is found in heated or aged cannabis. Medicinal benefits include pain relief, anti-inflammation, bone stimulant, and inhibition of cell growth in certain cancer.

Common Plant Terpenes

The following is an abbreviated list of scent chemicals that are found in cannabis and other flowering plants. There are hundreds of terpenes in cannabis and flowering plants.

Camphene has the aroma of fir needles. It may help reduce cardiovascular disease.

Carene smells sweet and pungent and can be found in juniper berries. It is a central nervous system relaxant.

Caryophyllene has a strong citrus smell and activates CB receptors. It is found in bay leaves, black pepper, cloves, and cinnamon. Medical uses include inhibition of cancer tumor growth, anti-anxiety, anti-depressant, and addiction treatment. Caryophyllene binds to peripheral CB2 receptors in the skin and can be used as an anti-inflammatory topically.

Geraniol has a sweet smell like roses and shows promise in neuropathy treatment.

Humulene is found in hops and works to reduce nausea and as an anti-tumor, anti-bacterial, anti-inflammatory, and appetite suppressant.

Limonene gives the aroma of lemons, limes, and oranges. Medicinal uses include increasing focus and attention, enhanced mood, gastrointestinal function improvement, ant-bacterial, and anti-fungal.

Linalool is found in lavender and has floral notes. Medicinal uses include sleep aid, anxiety and depression relief, and increased immune function.

Myrcene has a musky, earthy, herbal aroma found in mango, lemongrass, and thyme. It is a potent pain killer, anti-inflammatory, and anti-biotic. Myrcene is known to enhance the psychoactive effects of cannabinoids.

Terpineol is found in lilacs and has calming and relaxing effects. Terpineol is an acne inhibitor and works to boost antioxidants.

Terpinolene has a combination of pine and floral notes. Health benefits include drowsiness, allowing it to function as a sleep aid.

Pinene smells like pine needles and is found in rosemary, basil, and parsley. Health benefits include anti-inflammation, bronchodilation, alertness, and memory retention.

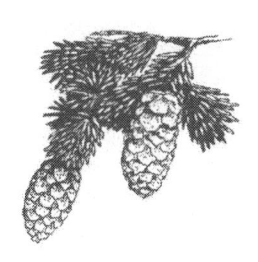

Medical Uses for Cannabis

The following is an abbreviated list of uses for cannabis. To see a list of conditions and cannabis effectiveness, strain, dosage, and method please see *The Cannabis Health Index* by Uwe Blesching or *The Cannabis Pharmacy* by Michael Backes.

- Addiction
- Acne
- Alzheimer's & Dementia
- ALS
- Anxiety
- Arthritis
- Asthma
- ADHD
- Autism
- AIDS
- Appetite
- Bipolar
- Cancer
- Chron's
- Depression
- Diabetes
- Tourette's
- Endometriosis
- Glaucoma
- Fibromyalgia
- IBS
- Hepatitis C
- Huntington's
- Insomnia
- Menopause
- Migraines
- MS
- Nausea
- Neuropathy
- Osteoporosis
- Pain
- Parkinson's
- Trauma
- Seizures

Biological Chemistry: Metabolism

Many factors cause our body to absorb and react to cannabis differently. Most people find CBD to have a relaxing effect. However, some people react to it like a cup of coffee. In some ways, it can be related to how Adderall calms people with ADHD but makes *normal* people have an energy rush. Our metabolism, diet, and environment change the chemical reactions in our body and how we may react to cannabis. What we eat, when we eat. and how we feel all factor in to how we can absorb cannabis. More importantly, we each have a different biochemistry or metabolism. Our individual biological chemistry is based on our genetics and changes throughout life. We inherit genes that have been switched on or off and can be prone to certain disease and illness. Children with ADHD, diabetes, epilepsy, or cancer are born with hereditary imbalances in their biological chemistry. Many diseases take time to develop. People can suffer minor imbalances with the onset of physical or mental illness developing later in life. Imbalances within our body and DNA can be positively changed with healthy lifestyle changes.

Our digestion process is something most of us take for granted. We have organisms in our digestive tract that keep us healthy when we provide them with the right nutrients and environment. Gut bacteria breaks down amino acids that regulate organ function, and affect our immune system, neurons, and mood. There are thousands of microbes that play an important role in immune system function. An imbalanced diet and gut can lead to autoimmune disease, asthma, irritable bowel syndrome (IBS), ulcerative colitis, autism, diabetes, rheumatoid arthritis, cancer, obesity, inflammation, MS, and neurodegenerative disease. The gut and brain are connected and communicate through biochemical signaling via the central nervous system or gut-brain axis.

Our diet works to sustain organ function. Conscious consumption and balanced diet are essential for healthy living. The organs within our cells and microbiota in our gut cannot function without oxygen, water, carbohydrates, lipids, protein, balanced pH, vitamins and phytonutrients. An imbalance in diet leads to imbalance in our mind and body.

Our metabolism encompasses all the chemical reactions our body needs to survive. While metabolism is commonly associated with the intake of food, it has more to do with energy needed for basic functions like keeping the heart beating. Our metabolism is affected by diet, exercise, stress, and genetic makeup. Exercise is important for muscle tone and bone health, but it uses little of our daily intake of calories.

Our greatest control is over what we choose to eat and drink. Essential fatty acids, antioxidants, and certain foods can increase the bioavailability of cannabinoids. Antioxidants have a network effect and work better together. The healthier food we combine while eating, the better we function and feel.

There are numerous interactions that effect how plant nutrients are absorbed. We each have a unique metabolism, making it hard to suggest a standard dose, delivery method, or strain. Our individual metabolism also changes throughout the day. The best approach to using cannabis is to follow the general guidelines in this manual and self-experiment responsibly.

Using Cannabis

All medicine typically needs to be taken regularly for patients to be able to determine the effects. CBD has a cumulative effect and can take up to three weeks of regular use before noticing results. While 10mg on its own may have no effect, over a period of weeks it will build up. CBD has a half-life of 24 hours, meaning that if you take 10mg one day that there will be 5mg in your system the next day. THC can take up to three days before being completely eliminated from your body.

During first time use, there can be little to no high. For people that try smoking, it may be as simple as not inhaling properly. After trying a few times, some people may not be aware of feeling a difference, but those around them will notice a more relaxed and happy state of being. It's difficult to determine how altered you may be if you have a lack of experience and awareness with mind-altering substances.

For the first few times, it is best to limit THC to between 1 to 5mg. CBD-rich and products high in other cannabinoids are non-psychoactive for most users and can be taken up to 20mg. Users may feel more relaxed or stimulated, but there is no high associated with CBD. Test for any sedating, stimulating, or mind-altering effects with new cannabis products in a comfortable space with enough time to experience effects uninterrupted.

There is no standard dose, delivery method, length of use, or variety of cannabis to find the optimal dose. It is up to each user to use their intuition and self-experiment to discover what dose, method, and strain works best.

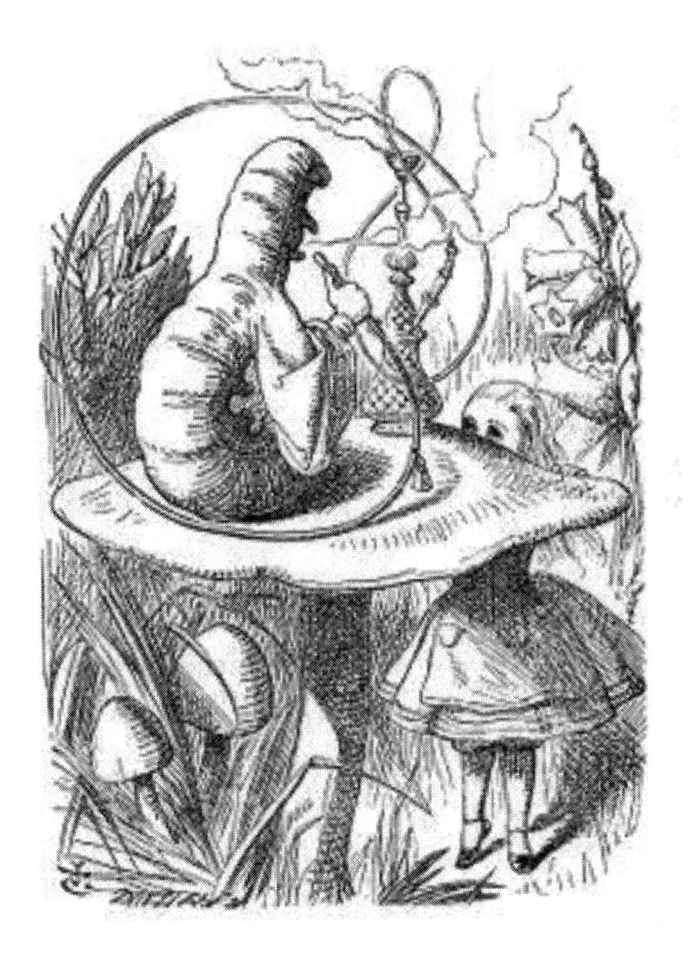

Choosing Medicine

It can be hard to know what to use when new to cannabis. With so many various products to choose from, it takes some experience, practice, and intuition to find what works best. Knowing what effect, you're looking to achieve helps to choose what medicine to use. People helping to sell products at cannabis dispensaries can vary in their education, experience, and knowledge of products. Not all companies describe their manufacturing practices in detail. By learning as a consumer about the active ingredients in cannabis, differences in dosing, and methods of consumption, it allows patients to know what to expect and tailor products to fit your needs. Remember this simple formula to help you determine the effect of any cannabis product:

Active Ingredients + Dosing + Method = Effect

The active ingredients of cannabis products are the plant chemicals or phytocannabinoids and terpenes. Dosing is determined by the number of milligrams of cannabinoid consumed. The method is the form you choose to use. Cannabis medicine comes in various forms including pre-rolled joints, lotions, oils, tea, and brownies. Cannabinoids are metabolized differently in the body depending on what form you choose to use.

The effects vary in how long it takes to feel the onset, intensity, and duration.

Ratios help determine the possible level of psychoactivity or high. A higher CBD-to-THC ratio lowers the risk of psychoactivity. Starting at a high CBD ratio and gradually increasing the amount of THC is suggested for new users looking to avoid altering their state of mind.

Manufactured products (anything other than cannabis flowers) can be processed with either whole cannabis plant or refined cannabis oil. Whole plant cannabis products are more effective and easier to dose as part of holistic plant therapy.

When using cannabis medicine regularly to regain or maintain health and wellness, many people wonder how to make it more effective. Cannabis can be enhanced with other medicine or activities. If using during the day, certain forms or cannabinoids can leave people feeling relaxed, focused, and energized with little psychoactivity. Cannabis strains high in pinene and limonene can be used with black tea, yerba mate, or coffee to enhance the stimulating effects. At night, cannabis high in linalool and terpinolene can be taken with melatonin, valerian root, or chamomile tea to enhance the sedating effects. Cannabis high in myrcene and carene can be taken with kava, ashwagandha, and rishi to enhance creativity, stress relief and euphoria. Cannabis high in caryophyllene and terpineol can be taken with chocolate, blueberries, ginger, or cumin to enhance the antioxidant and anti-inflammatory effects. Cannabis strains can be tailored and paired with other medicine to better reach the desired effect.

When purchasing any cannabis product for consumption, there are certain quality standards to ensure safety. Legal dispensaries ensure that the plants were grown organically and processed without contamination or additives.

Dosing

All medicine is highly individualized and the methods for dosing cannabis vary. Two people using the same strain or cannabis product can experience two different effects. Whole plant medicine (and pharmaceuticals) have a range of dosages and are not on-size-fits-all. Patients with the same condition can respond differently to medicine, even when using the same method, strain, and dosage. Each person has a unique biochemistry, endocannabinoid system, and DNA that respond differently to cannabis.

Safely and successfully experiment with the many options available by using observation to gauge your physical and mental reactions. Keeping a journal of plant use helps find the optimal method and dose. Most patients find it doesn't take much to feel at ease. During intense recovery, some patients might take higher doses at first to regain balance. Once health and harmony are established, micro and moderate dosing can be used as prevention and maintenance. It can be helpful for users to cut back or abstain periodically to maintain balance if using cannabis regularly.

Finding the optimal dose to experience relief from symptoms is a bit like Goldilocks and the Three Bears. Take too little, and you'll feel little to no effect (and still be uncomfortable). Take too much, and you can become uncomfortable from anxiety, lethargy, paranoia, or dry mouth. You will find comfort and relief using *just* the right amount.

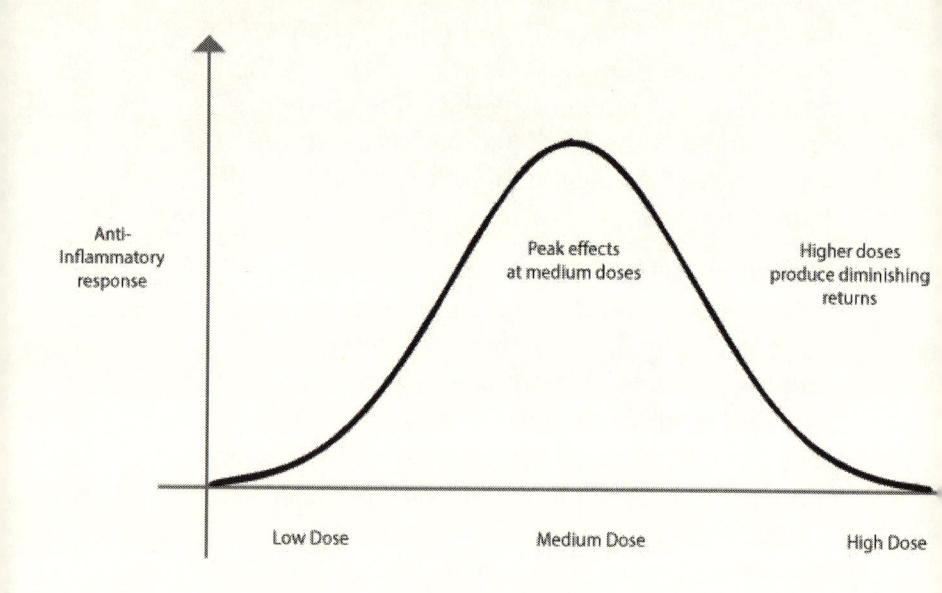

[Figure: Bell curve showing anti-inflammatory response vs. dose. Y-axis: Anti-Inflammatory response. X-axis: Low Dose, Medium Dose, High Dose. Labels: "Peak effects at medium doses" at the top of the curve, "Higher doses produce diminishing returns" on the right side.]

Starting low and going slow when dosing is the best suggested method to find the optimal amount of medicine. Start with low doses of THC and CBD and only increase the dose after a few days or weeks of use. This method, called titration, prevents intense psychoactivity, decreases side-effects, and prevents building tolerance. Users clearly establish a dose that helps relieve stress and pain without ever going overboard. Large or macro-doses are better suited for experienced users with chronic or terminal illnesses. The worst thing that can happen when "over-dosing" is lethargy, nausea, and dysphoria for up to eight hours. Some people find the experience so unpleasant that they become unwilling to use cannabis again. Some cannabis users require an intense amount of medicine while others look to use as little as possible. Sustaining an intense effect may take increasingly large doses. Patients needing a clinical dose, but wary of feeling high, rely on building a tolerance to the psychoactive qualities of cannabinoids through titration.

Micro-dosing can be effective for creativity, energy, focus, insomnia, recovery from exercise, headaches, euphoria, anxiety, mild pain, and basic metabolic or blood sugar disorders. A micro-dose is generally one to two milligrams but can be up to ten milligrams for experienced users. It allows users to have a sense of balance without the buzz.

Standard or moderate doses aid with inflammation, depression, moderate pain, menstrual cramps, autoimmune disease, gastrointestinal disorders, neurodegenerative disease, heart disease, seizures, migraines, and autism. A standard dose is generally between five to twenty-five milligrams.

Macro-dosing is used clinically to treat epilepsy, severe addiction, cancer, liver disease, severe pain, post-traumatic stress, organ failure, and life-threatening conditions. A macro-dose is typically anything over fifty milligrams. Some patients use upwards of one thousand milligrams a day.

Methods of Consumption

Our body absorbs medicine differently depending on the variety, method, dose, metabolism, mood, and level of pain. When it comes to method of consumption, there are variables in the amount of time it takes to feel the effect (onset), the amount of time the effect lasts (duration), and the number of cannabinoids that are available into the bloodstream (bioavailability). The metabolism of cannabinoids is a dynamic process, can change as we age, and can be affected by frequency and dosage[3].

The more serious the illness, the more methods or therapies should be used to restore balance. Systemic issues such as nerve pain can be treated via the bloodstream with a tincture or edible for recurring pain, vaporization for acute pain, and externally with topicals. For example, a person with trouble sleeping could use vaporization to feel sleepy, a tincture to fall asleep, and an edible to stay asleep all night long.

Research has shown a large variability in bioavailability of cannabinoids when smoking

---

[3] Huestis, Marilyn A. "Human cannabinoid pharmacokinetics" *Chemistry & biodiversity* vol. 4,8 (2007): 1770-804.

cannabis, even while controlling the length of inhalation, hold time, exhalation time, and time between puffs. That means we all absorb different amount of cannabis. Diet plays an important role in bioavailability. Beta-caryophyllene, omegas, and other chemicals can be found in our diet that interacts with the ECS. Certain foods increase the bioavailability of THC and cannabinoids.

Plant medicine is commonly infused into chocolate. Humans have used cacao as the primary remedy or vehicle to deliver other medicine since 460 AD. Raw cacao provides anandamide, antioxidants, and acts as support for enhanced absorption with exceptional amounts of magnesium, copper, zinc, iron, Vitamin C, omega-6, fiber, and chromium[4]. As one of the most medicinally beneficial plants, it's a shame that not all chocolate is sourced and processed the same. Poverty, salve and child-labor take place in countries that produce cacao. An estimated 2.1 million West African children work in dangerous conditions[5]. Please buy fair-trade or ethically sourced organic chocolate. Non-organic products are treated heavily with pesticides, fungicides, and may have GMOs

---

[4] Katz, David L et al. "Cocoa and chocolate in human health and disease *"Antioxidants & redox signaling* vol. 15,10 (2011): 2779-811.
[5] Brain O'Keefe, "Inside Big Chocolate's Child Labor Problem," *Fortune,* March 1, 2016, fortune.com/big-chocolate-child-labor

added. Furthermore, chocolate is commonly Dutch-processed to reduce bitterness and provide a rich-color. Unfortunately, this also eliminates many of the antioxidant benefits. Cacao helps prevent diabetes but eating too many milk chocolate bars leads to weight gain.

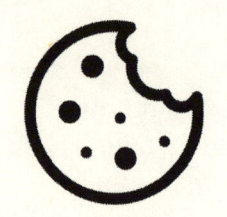

Edible

Edibles are processed through the liver and convert into a more psychoactive and sedative Delta-11 THC. Edibles can hit stronger when taken on an empty stomach. Raw cannabis that is non-psychoactive can decarboxylate if your stomach is full of food. Micro-dosing gives most users a functional high. Increasing the dose leads to increased psychoactivity, dry mouth, and possible negative side effects like paranoia and lethargy. Terpenes are mostly lost during cooking or manufactured using distillates. Edibles can be labeled as *Sativa* or *Indica* as a marketing gimmick.

> Directions: Eat a little. Wait 2 hours. Eat a little more if not noticeable effects.
>
> Onset: Digestion slows down when consuming edibles creating an onset time between 1 and 2 hours[6].
>
> Duration: 6 to 8 hours
>
> Bioavailability: Varies between 4-20%

---

[6] McCallum RW et al. "Delta-9-tetrahydrocannabinol delays the gastric emptying of solid food in humans: a double-blind, randomized study." *Aliment Pharmacol Ther.* 1999 Jan;13(1):77-80.

Sublingual Tincture

Tinctures are made with alcohol and have a higher absorption rate than edibles. Oil-based tinctures are useful for users looking to avoid alcohol, but are mostly processed like an edible. Oils high in omegas, such as MCT or olive oil, can be partially absorbed under the tongue if left for 3-10 minutes. With alcohol tinctures, cannabinoids and terpenes are quickly transported to the brain through the carotid artery from glands and ducts under the tongue. Alcohol tinctures can be diluted with water to avoid the burning sensation.

Directions: Drop under the tongue or cheek.

Onset: Immediate to 15 minutes with tinctures. Up to two hours with oils.

Duration: 4 and 6 hours

Bioavailability: 40%

Topical

Topicals are salves, oils, bath salts, or lotions applied directly to the skin for local relief. Topicals are non-psychoactive and do not create a head-trip or high. THC does not show up on a blood or urine test[7]. Cannabinoid molecules are large and do not pass through skin cells. They interact with CB and TRP[8] receptors in skin cells, glands, immune cells, and nerve endings to stimulate endocannabinoid homeostasis. Cannabinoids suppress the expression of diseased cells and treat psoriasis. They also promote apoptosis in cancer cells and modulate tumor growth[9]. THC, THCA, CBD, CBDA, CBG, CBC, and CBN are effective for pain relief, neuropathy, inflammation. skin disorders, acne, menstrual relief, and burns[10]. Terpenes or

---

[7] C. Hess et al. "Topical application of THC containing products is not able to find positive cannabinoid finding in blood or urine" *Forensic Science International* vol 272 (2017): 68-71

[8] Caterina, Michael J. "TRP channel cannabinoid receptors in skin sensation, homeostasis, and inflammation" *ACS chemical neuroscience* vol. 5,11 (2014): 1107-16.

[9] Casanova M. L. et al. (2003) Inhibition of skin tumor growth and angiogenesis in vivo by activation of cannabinoid receptors. J. Clin. Invest. 111, 43–50.

[10] Pucci M. et al. (2011) Endocannabinoid signaling and epidermal differentiation. Eur. J. Dermatol 21(Suppl 2), 29

essential oils are smaller molecules and pass through with ease. Topicals can be infused with synergistic herbs to enhance the properties and effects of cannabis. Cannabis roots are highly useful in topical because they are high in terpenes with anti-inflammatory properties.

Directions: Apply where needed for relief. Covering the skin with a non-permeable substance, or applying after a shower, helps increases effectiveness.

Onset: Immediate relief

Duration: 4 to 6 hours

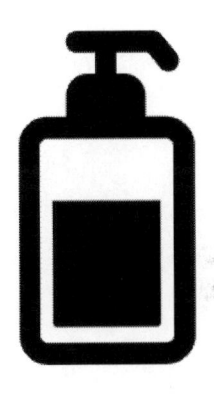

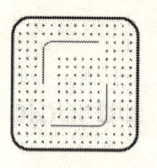

Transdermal

Transdermal patches are intended to be used on the skin and disperse a steady amount of medication throughout the day. Transdermal patches and topical products only work if the molecules are small enough to enter the bloodstream. Chemical enhancers or microneedles are added in pharmaceutical-grade patches to allow macromolecules like cannabinoids to enter the bloodstream through the skin. Current transdermal patches do not have enhancers or microneedles. No large-scale study on the effectiveness of transdermal patches is currently available. Most patches works as a topical. Reported benefits of patches include quick relief, long-lasting effects, high bioavailability, and controlled dosing.

>Onset: 15 minutes
>
>Duration: Up to 12 hours
>
>Bioavailability: Unknown

Vaporization & Smoking

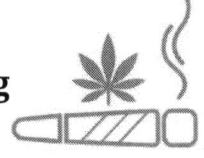

Vaporizing exposes users to fewer toxins than smoke and reduces many health risks associated with combustion[11]. Smoking cannabis has not been shown to increase the risk of cancer. In fact, it does the opposite and works as a protectant from cancer. It also increases the availability of cannabinoids. Ultimately, temperature determines the cannabinoid to by-product ratio and compounds released[12]. The benefits of inhaling plant medicine by smoking or vaporizing include immediate relief, increased effectiveness, and controlled dosing.

Onset: Immediate

Duration: 1 to 2 hours

Bioavailability: Varies between 10-35%

---

[11] Earleywine M, Barnwell SS. "Decreased respiratory symptoms in cannabis users who vaporize." *Harm Reduction J*. 2007 Apr 16;4-11.

[12] Pomahacova B, et al. "Cannabis smoke condensate III: the cannabinoid content of vaporised Cannabis sativa." *Inhalation Toxicology*. 2009. Nov;21(13):1108-12.

Suppositories

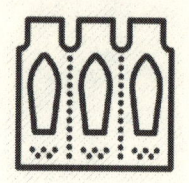

Suppositories are a good option for patients who have trouble keeping food down or are looking to avoid smoking. Users suffering endometritis, prostate or rectal cancer, menstrual cramps, hemorrhoids, and gastrointestinal disorders find localized and systemic relief. Bioavailability is unknown and more research needs to be done.

> Directions: Insert just far enough to keep in as pushing it up too far can lead to increased liver absorption and high-psychoactivity.
>
> Onset: 15 minutes to 1 hour
>
> Duration: 4 to 6 hours

Growing

Growing cannabis plants is easy to do if you understand the basics of gardening. As a *weed* it takes very little sunlight, nutrients, and water to survive. The sky is the limit when given proper care. Outdoor cannabis plants grown in nutrient-rich soil with direct sunlight and regular watering can grow over 12-feet tall. As an annual plant, cannabis goes through a vegetative growth period during twelve hours of sunlight or more, and flowers when there is less than twelve hours of light. The bigger the container they are in, the bigger they will grow. A 3-gallon or 5-gallon pot works for keeping the plants under 6' tall. Topping, cutting, or pinching off the top part of the plant can also help control the plant height.

Most states allow six mature cannabis plants. Germinating seeds takes 1-2 weeks. Paper towels can be used to sprout seeds. Move seeds into soil and give lots of sunlight for 2-3 weeks. The vegetative growth takes place from April-June, or 2-8 weeks indoors and high amounts of nitrogen help. Flowering takes 6-8 weeks for cannabis plants, and high amounts of phosphorous.

The main nutrients required to grow any plant are N-P-K or nitrogen, phosphorous, and potassium. Plants also require calcium, magnesium, and sulfur. If the soil used to grow cannabis is lacking these main nutrients, any plant will die shortly after sprouting. Micronutrients are necessary to help the plant survive and produce flowers. Balance is key when fertilizing and watering. An imbalance in soil pH, water, or fertilizer limits plant growth. Cannabis seedlings or clones do better in high humidity with temperatures between 68-77ºF. Mature plants do better with drier air and cooler or warmer weather. When possible, cannabis plants should be kept from frost, high humidity, rain, and extreme heat. Going over 85 ºF can slow plant growth.

Watering and fertilizing can be a bit tricky when you don't know what to look for. Leaves should be dark green (not yellowing or spotted) and rigid. If you're not sure how moist the soil is, then simply stick your finger in a few inches to check for dryness. Plants with wilted leaves or dry soil need water. Depending on the size, weather, and type of growth, plants may need to be watered anywhere from every day to every three days. Over-watering stunts plant growth and can cause the roots to rot.

Organic fertilizer must be used when growing cannabis. If you are unsure of the quality of the soil you are growing in, then using pots ensures the plants don't absorb toxins. Many organically enriched soils are easily available and affordable. Natural sources of fertilizer can be used such as compost tea, coffee grounds, tea bags, leaves, bat guano, manure, and mycorrhizae. Plants always grow better when in healthy soil full of microbes. Giving the right amount of nutrients allows you to have the biggest yield possible with potent flowers.

Pruning the lower branches of your plants allows the nutrients to flow into other parts of the plant. Lower branches also receive less sunlight and produce fewer flowers, so removing them is a good idea. Plants should be pruned enough to allow for good air flow in order to prevent mold or powdery mildew. It is much easier to prevent a problem than to try and regain control. Adding nematodes to the soil can easily be done and helps manage pests. If problems such as aphids or spider mites occur, then releasing ladybugs or praying mantis can resolve the problem. Remember to never use any fungicides or pesticides.

Harvesting & Curing Cannabis

Growing cannabis is only part of the process. Curing means drying and storing cannabis in order to maintain the smell and effect. There are many ways to harvest and cure cannabis.

Harvesting and curing cannabis can entirely change the smell and effects for better or worse. When done incorrectly, cannabis has little effect and smells like hay. You have the ability to influence the overall effect by choosing when to harvest. During the final weeks of flowering, cannabis trichomes change in color. Using a magnifying glass makes it easy to see the tiny hairs develop a bulb and change from clear to milky to amber.

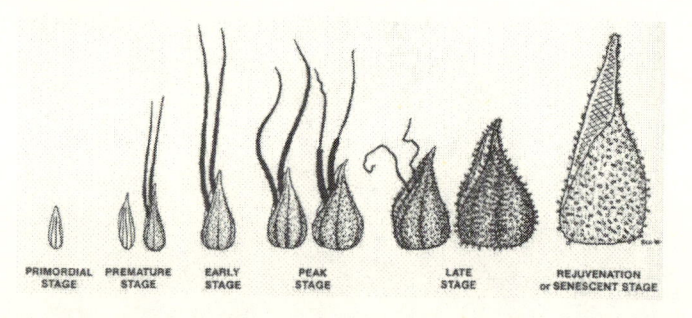

PRIMORDIAL STAGE — PREMATURE STAGE — EARLY STAGE — PEAK STAGE — LATE STAGE — REJUVENATION or SENESCENT STAGE

Harvesting the plant can be done in countless ways. Some people choose to harvest all at once, while others cut down branches as they ripen. Harvesting early typically provides a more cerebral effect. "Sativa" users may want to harvest their uplifting strains earlier. As the trichomes turn amber, effects typically become more relaxing and sedative. You can harvest with only a portion of the trichomes amber—or all of them. Be careful not to harvest your plant too early, as it will not have enough time to develop terpenes and cannabinoids.

The most popular way to harvest cannabis is by cutting down branches, pulling off big leaves, and hanging them on a wire. A slower cure produces higher quality medicine. Cannabis should be dried in a dark room with temperatures between 60-70ºF and a humidity of 45-55%. Using a fan helps to circulate the air and prevent mold. Drying can take anywhere from five to fifteen days, depending on the size of the branch. You can check to see if the flowers are ready to be stored by trying to snap the branch. If a branch bends, then there is still too much moisture in the flower. Wait until the branch breaks cleanly apart before storing, but do not over-dry plants.

Once cannabis is finished drying, the curing process continues for another three to six weeks. If you haven't manicured the cannabis during the harvesting process, then it is good to do so before jarring the flowers. Place the trimmed buds into light-resistant airtight glass jars. Seal the jars and store them in a cool place. After a day, you should notice some moisture return to the outer part of the bud. If not, the flower was over-dried. If there is the smell of ammonia, then the flower wasn't dry enough when jarred. During the first week, it is important to "burp" the jar or allow moisture to escape and circulate the air. After the first week, you will only need to open the jars every other day. Be sure to always store cannabis in a cool place out of sunlight.

Crafting Cannabis

Quality cannabis flower results in quality medicine when made under the right conditions. It can be cheaper to purchase flower and make your own tinctures, topical, and edibles that are more potent than what you can buy in stores. Certain methods of production maintain the complex full spectrum found in raw cannabis flower. Cannabis is non-psychoactive until heated. Cannabinoids undergo chemical changes over time when exposed to light and heat. Decarboxylation is the process of adding heat to cannabis to activate different components. Chemical composition and effect vary depending on the length of time and heat added to the plant. To activate the highest number of cannabinoids, heat cannabis flower in a covered glass baking dish for thirty minutes at 250ºF and leave to cool before processing. By heating cannabis at a lower temperature, it takes more time but preserves more terpenes and cannabinoids. The ways of growing, processing, and crafting cannabis are limitless.

Homogenization is the process of continual mixing to evenly distribute medicine. It takes a bit of chemistry and creativity to be able to homogenize cannabis into a fat source. Cannabinoids don't dissolve in water—they need fat.

Simple Recipes

Cannabis can be crafted or manufactured using different methods. Low heat allows for a slower infusion process. High heat speeds up the process but requires more care and concentration. Cold-processed cannabis provides an array of health benefits without the psychoactivity or high.

The following recipes are able to be modified. You can add more or use less cannabis depending on the desired potency. Cannabis flower have a stronger potency than the leaves. You can grade the potency based on the amount of sticky hairs. Shake or trim will vary in potency depending on the amount of trichomes present. The stem, leaves, flowers, and roots of the cannabis plant have different medicinal properties. Remember that whole plant infusions create more medicinally beneficial results.

Cannabis Oil

Oil can be used in cooking, baking, or added to beverages. You can also add beeswax and other herbs to the oil and create a topical, or simply apply the oil directly to your skin. Oil can also be mixed with Epsom salts and used in the bath.

Ingredients:

- 1 cup cold-pressed organic olive, avocado, grapeseed, sunflower, sesame, macadamia, or safflower oil
- 10 grams ground cannabis
- 1 tablespoon organic lecithin (optional)

Equipment:

- Glass jar
- Cheesecloth

Instructions:

- Decarboxylate cannabis if desired.
- Fill jar with cannabis and cover with oil.
- Store out of sunlight in a cool place for 4-6 weeks. Shake every 3 days.
- Strain. Store in dark glass bottle.

Crockpot method:

- Decarboxylate cannabis if desired.
- Fill crockpot with cannabis and cover with oil. Add lecithin.
- Keep crockpot on warm (at 160ºF) for 8-12 hours, stirring every half-hour.
- Strain. Store in dark glass bottle.

Cannabis Tincture

Ingredients:

- 1 cup grain alcohol (151 or 190 proof)
- 10 grams ground cannabis
- Cheesecloth

Equipment:

- Glass jar
- Caution as alcohol is highly flammable.

Instructions:

- Decarboxylate cannabis if desired.
- Fill glass jar up to ¾ full of cannabis. Cover so alcohol is two inches above the herb.
- Store out of sunlight in a cool 4-6 weeks. Shake twice a day for one month.
- Strain through cheesecloth into dark glass bottle.
- Dilute with distilled water (if desired)

Full Extract Cannabis Oil (Rick Simpson Oil)

Rich Simpson oil is the common name for concentrated cannabis oil used mostly in cancer treatment. Full extract oil is the most concentrated form of cannabis you can make at home, and is used to treat serious medical conditions. Children with seizures typically use CBD-rich oils. Concentrated oils have a very long shelf life and can be used by placing directly on the gums (or buy empty capsules to make your own pills).

Instructions: Hazardous—Use caution!

- Slowly heat 1-5 cups of ethanol cannabis in a crockpot. Do not use an open flame. Warm or lowest setting for 30-45 minutes per cup of alcohol, constantly stirring until it becomes a sticky syrup. Cool for one minute and quickly pour into a dark glass bottle. Cook in a well-ventilated area.

Cannabis Suppositories

Ingredients:

- 1/2 cup organic fair-trade coco butter
- 1/2 gram Full-Extract Cannabis Oil

Equipment:

- Double boiler
- Silicone Mini Ice Cube Tray

Instructions:

- Melt cocoa butter in double boiler
- Mix in cannabis oil and stir to evenly distribute medicine.
- Pour into mold. Cool in fridge. Store in glass container.
- Store in the fridge until ready for use. Cocoa butter melts on skin contact and is too soft to insert at room temperature.

Cautions

Cannabis is non-toxic, and no lethal dose has ever occurred. No brain or organ damage has been reported in studies. Long-term exposure to cannabis does not cause persistent cognitive deficits nor schizophrenia in adults. CB receptors do not control breathing and heart rate as opioids do.

THC causes an increased heart rate of 20-50bpm. Patients with heart conditions and on prescription medicine should discuss cannabis use with their doctor. An overdose cannot kill you but can cause adverse reaction and possibly a feeling of panic. When over-stimulated, the ECS can trigger or worsen the symptom that would otherwise be relieved when using the optimal dose. Unnecessary stress can be avoided through micro-dosing.

THCA and CBD are commonly said to be non-psychoactive. Most users report no change in behavior. However, a minority of users' experience CBD similar to caffeine. Symptoms reported include hyperactivity, diarrhea, and restlessness. Macro doses produce sedating effects. Test new cannabis products in small amounts for sensitivity. All side-effects from cannabis can be resolved with changes in delivery method, ratio, variety, or dosing.

As cannabis absorbs fungicides, herbicides, and insecticides, it is best to test for purity to avoid cancer, skin irritation, neurologic disorders, reproductive problems, and other disorders. Conscious practices and lab testing ensure the final product is free of pesticides, toxins, heavy metals, containments, pests, mold and mildew. Contaminated medicine may be toxic, especially to patients with a compromised immune system.

Using products that have high levels of toxins or residual solvents can cause hyperemesis or an allergic and possibly severe reaction to contaminated medicine. Symptoms include headache and vomiting. Solvents used to manufacture cannabis products and concentrates can be made using carcinogenic neurotoxins such as butane, propane, or hexane. Growing your own cannabis allows you to control the environment, for the most part. Any cannabis product purchased at a licensed dispensary has been lab tested. Concentrating contaminated plant matter increases the risk of side effects. Concentrates and vape cartridges can contain added toxic substances, additives, or thinners with unknown long-term effects. Solvents and toxic additives can lead to headaches, nervous system depression, nausea, dizziness, and other possible adverse side effects when consumed. Pure cannabis oil is the safest product to vaporize. Any side effect can be eliminated by eliminating product use.

Driving

New users driving under the influence of THC have a lack of tracking ability, attentiveness, judgment, peripheral vision, and coordination. Driving should be avoided for up to eight hours. Many users report a heightened sense of focus while using cannabis and joke about being attentive for police. Under mild-to-moderate doses of THC, most drivers still over-compensate, can be easily distracted, or react slower than normal.

Alcohol

It is not advised to mix cannabis and alcohol. Edibles are processed through the liver and should be avoided with alcohol. Coordination and extreme disorientation are possible as alcohol increases the absorption of THC.

Pregnancy & Nursing

Cannabis use in pregnant women is socially frowned upon. Instead of using cannabis medicine during labor, many women receive an epidural without realizing it's a synthetic derivative of cocaine with potential negative side-effects. There has been no evidence of difference in growth of the fetus or development of the newborn for cannabis-using mothers[13]. In

---

[13] D. M. Fergusson, et al., "Maternal Use of Cannabis and Pregnancy Outcome," *BLOG: An International Journal of Obstetrics and Gynaecology* 109 (2002): 21-27

fact, the ECS is involved in regulating many of the chemical messengers in fertility and breastfeeding. For women with naturally low levels of anandamide, CBD can help increase the possibility of pregnancy. This does not mean pregnant and nursing mothers should use cannabis heavily. Exercise, massage, stretching, and a balanced diet before, during, and after pregnancy should be the priority. Nausea and excess stress from tension in mothers can cause harm on the fetus. Excess weight loss from morning sickness can lead to malnutrition.

Every patient needs to weigh the benefits with possible risks and avoid any possible harm by using cannabis sparingly and in small amounts to decrease nausea and pain. Breast milk contains endocannabinoids and will carry phytocannabinoids, as well. Cannabis can be used to replace missing cannabinoids in the breastmilk of postpartum mothers.

Children and Minors

A balanced and functioning ECS is critical for development. CBD, THCA, and cannabinoids other than THC are recommended for people twenty-one and under. The benefits of using cannabinoid medicine under supervision and in moderation far outweighs the risks[14]. Children

---

[14] Melanie C. Dreher, Kevin Nugent, Rebekah Hudgins, "Prenatal Marijuana Exposure and Neonatal Outcomes in Jamaica: An Ethnographic Study" *Pediatrics* 93, no. 2 (1994): 254-260.

with autism, ADHD, cancer, diabetes, seizures, and Tourette syndrome have all found relief without the side effects associated with pharmaceuticals. Mild and moderate cannabis use doesn't show negative long-term effects. Heavy use can lead to psychological dependency depending on environmental, familial, and economic factors.

For healthy children and minors in a stable and nurturing environment, it is important that they limit the use of any drug during brain development. Pets and children should generally receive medicine that is high in CBD and low in THC. However, doctors have reported that, under supervision, certain children responded better to THC.

Pharmaceutical Interactions

If taking any prescription drug, you should investigate if there are possible interactions with cannabis and speak with your doctor prior to using plant medicine. While there isn't much risk of a drug-drug interaction, certain drugs may require a smaller dose when using cannabis[15]. CBD can increase or decrease the breakdown of other medication.[16]

---

[15] Alexandra L. Geffrey, et al., "Drug-drug Interaction between Clobazam and Cannabidiol in Children with Refractory Epilepsy," *Epilepsia* 56, no. 8 (2015): 1246-1251.

[16] K. Watanabe, et al., "Cytochrome P450 Enzymes Involved in the Metabolim of Tetrahydrocannabinols and Cannabinol by

RX interactions are noted in the following drugs, although this is not a complete list: AEDs, steroids, Ca channel blockers, antihistamines, prokinetics, HIV antiviral, immune modulators, benzodiazepines, anti-arrhythmic, antibiotics, antipsychotics, antidepressants, anti-ecliptics, beta blockers, NSAIDs, and PPIs.

Drug Testing

Cannabinoids are excreted through feces and urine in approximately three to five days. Remnants can also be stored in the fatty tissue for regular users and take weeks to eliminate all traces of phytocannabinoids.

Smoking

Cannabinoids bind to the carcinogenic protein caused by combustion. There is no evidence of an increase in the incidence of cancers in the lungs, trachea, larynx, pharynx, and esophagus even in heavy smokers. The National Institute on Drug Abuse has funded several studies in efforts to find harm in smoking cannabis. Many studies ultimately found a slightly protective effect. Cells damaged by cannabis smoke and tar initiate apoptosis and die off.

While there is no conclusive evidence that smoking cannabis is detrimental; vaporization is considered a safer alternative.

Human Hepatic Microsomes," *Life Sciences* 80, no. 15 (2007): 1415-1419.

It allows users to avoid carcinogenic chemicals caused by combustion and tar, providing less irritation. Cannabinoids are bronchodilators and help bring in air to the lungs, so the benefits of using cannabis outweighs any risk.

Smudging is the burning of herbs and plants as a method of purification to balance the physical body and atmosphere. Ceremonies with smoke are used to carry thoughts and prayers into the spirit world. When we inhale smoke, we ourselves are thought to be cleansed as we embark on a journey to the spirit world and come back reborn. The science behind hot-boxing, secondhand smoke, and essential oil diffusers explains this phenomenon. When releasing smoke into the air, we inhale minimal amounts of the particulates. Certain smells cause us to feel relaxed, energized, hungry, or clear our sinuses. When releasing herbs with scent or psychoactive components, we inhale trace amounts and experience an effect.

Nicotine receptors share the same receptors as THC. Try a balanced ratio of CBD and THC, instead of the combination of tobacco and cannabis flower, if you tend to mix tobacco with cannabis.

Journals

The following pages can be used to help track cannabis use. Keeping a journal can be helpful for cannabis users to track the effects of different products, strains, or home-made remedies.

Journal 1

Date: _____ Time: _____

Dose: _____ Method: _____

Strain/Product: _____

Last Meal: ☐ Light ☐ Moderate ☐ Heavy
When: ☐ 1 hr ☐ 2 hrs ☐ 3+ hrs

Desired effect: ☐ Pain Relief ☐ Euphoria
☐ Relaxation ☐ Reduce cravings ☐ Appetite
☐ Focus ☐ Energy ☐ Creativity ☐ Sleep
☐ _____

Pain level: _____ Stress level: _____

0 1 2 3 4 5 6 7 8 9 10

Intensity Graph:

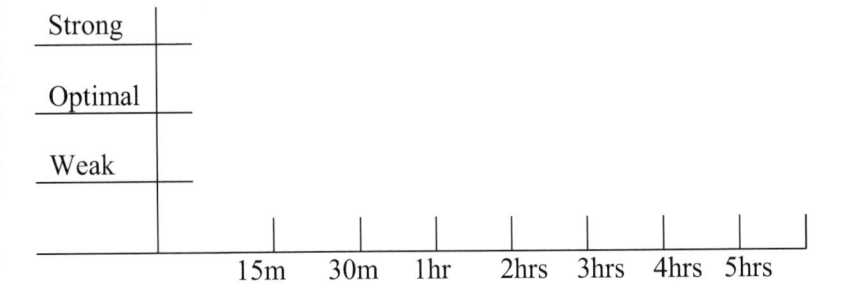

Strong

Optimal

Weak

15m 30m 1hr 2hrs 3hrs 4hrs 5hrs

Journal 1

Phytocannabinoids Used: ☐ THCA ☐ THC
☐ THCV ☐ CBD ☐ CBG ☐ CBC ☐ CBN
☐ CBDA   ☐ _____

Terpenes Used: ☐ Humulene ☐ Limonene
☐ Pinene ☐ Linalool ☐ Myrcene
☐ Terpinolene ☐ Geraneol ☐ Nerolidol
☐ Ocimene ☐ Terpineol
☐ _____

Diet: ☐ Beta-caryophyllene ☐ Anti-inflammatories
☐ Pro-biotics ☐ Omegas ☐ Adaptogens
☐ Antioxidants
☐ _____

Daily Activity: ☐ Light ☐ Moderate ☐ Intense

Experience:_____
_____
_____

Side Effects: ☐ Dry mouth ☐ Over-stimulated
☐ Drowsy ☐ Lethargic ☐ Paranoia
☐ _____

Desired Effect: ☐ Yes ☐ No ☐ _____

Rating: ★ ★ ★ ★ ★

Journal 2

Date: _____ Time: _____

Dose: _____ Method: _____

Strain/Product: _____

Last Meal: ☐ Light ☐ Moderate ☐ Heavy
When: ☐ 1 hr ☐ 2 hrs ☐ 3+ hrs

Desired effect: ☐ Pain Relief ☐ Euphoria
☐ Relaxation ☐ Reduce cravings ☐ Appetite
☐ Focus ☐ Energy ☐ Creativity ☐ Sleep
☐ _____

Pain level: _____ Stress level: _____

Intensity Graph:

	15m	30m	1hr	2hrs	3hrs	4hrs	5hrs
Strong							
Optimal							
Weak							

Journal 2

Phytocannabinoids Used: ☐ THCA ☐ THC
☐ THCV ☐ CBD ☐ CBG ☐ CBC ☐ CBN
☐ CBDA   ☐ _____

Terpenes Used: ☐ Humulene   ☐ Limonene
☐ Pinene   ☐ Linalool   ☐ Myrcene
☐ Terpinolene ☐ Geraneol   ☐ Nerolidol
☐ Ocimene ☐ Terpineol
☐ _____

Diet: ☐ Beta-caryophyllene ☐ Anti-inflammatories
☐ Pro-biotics ☐ Omegas ☐ Adaptogens
☐ Antioxidants
☐ _____

Daily Activity: ☐ Light   ☐ Moderate   ☐ Intense

Experience: _____
_____
_____

Side Effects: ☐ Dry mouth   ☐ Over-stimulated
☐ Drowsy ☐ Lethargic ☐ Paranoia
☐ _____

Desired Effect: ☐ Yes   ☐ No   ☐ _____

Rating: ★★★★★

Journal 3

Date: _____   Time: _____

Dose: _____   Method: _____

Strain/Product: _____

Last Meal: ☐ Light ☐ Moderate ☐ Heavy
When: ☐ 1 hr   ☐ 2 hrs   ☐ 3+ hrs

Desired effect: ☐ Pain Relief ☐ Euphoria
☐ Relaxation ☐ Reduce cravings ☐ Appetite
☐ Focus ☐ Energy ☐ Creativity ☐ Sleep
☐ _____

Pain level: _____   Stress level: _____

Intensity Graph:

Strong
Optimal
Weak

15m 30m 1hr 2hrs 3hrs 4hrs 5hrs

Journal 3

Phytocannabinoids Used: ☐ THCA ☐ THC
☐ THCV ☐ CBD ☐ CBG ☐ CBC ☐ CBN
☐ CBDA   ☐ _____

Terpenes Used: ☐ Humulene ☐ Limonene
☐ Pinene   ☐ Linalool ☐ Myrcene
☐ Terpinolene ☐ Geraneol ☐ Nerolidol
☐ Ocimene ☐ Terpineol
☐ _____

Diet: ☐ Beta-caryophyllene ☐ Anti-inflammatories
☐ Pro-biotics ☐ Omegas ☐ Adaptogens
☐ Antioxidants
☐ _____

Daily Activity: ☐ Light ☐ Moderate ☐ Intense

Experience: _____
_____
_____

Side Effects: ☐ Dry mouth ☐ Over-stimulated
☐ Drowsy ☐ Lethargic ☐ Paranoia
☐ _____

Desired Effect: ☐ Yes ☐ No ☐ _____

Rating: ★★★★★

Journal 4

Date: _____ Time: _____

Dose: _____ Method: _____

Strain/Product: _____

Last Meal: ☐ Light ☐ Moderate ☐ Heavy
When: ☐ 1 hr ☐ 2 hrs ☐ 3+ hrs

Desired effect: ☐ Pain Relief ☐ Euphoria
☐ Relaxation ☐ Reduce cravings ☐ Appetite
☐ Focus ☐ Energy ☐ Creativity ☐ Sleep
☐ _____

Pain level: _____ Stress level: _____

Intensity Graph:

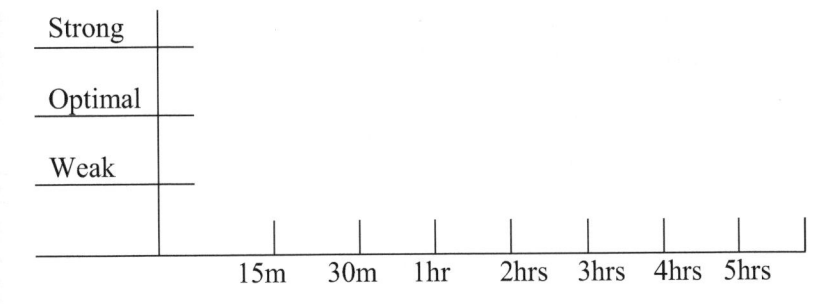

Strong	
Optimal	
Weak	

15m 30m 1hr 2hrs 3hrs 4hrs 5hrs

Journal 4

Phytocannabinoids Used: ☐ THCA ☐ THC
☐ THCV ☐ CBD ☐ CBG ☐ CBC ☐ CBN
☐ CBDA ☐ _____

Terpenes Used: ☐ Humulene ☐ Limonene
☐ Pinene ☐ Linalool ☐ Myrcene
☐ Terpinolene ☐ Geraneol ☐ Nerolidol
☐ Ocimene ☐ Terpineol
☐ _____

Diet: ☐ Beta-caryophyllene ☐ Anti-inflammatories
☐ Pro-biotics ☐ Omegas ☐ Adaptogens
☐ Antioxidants
☐ _____

Daily Activity: ☐ Light ☐ Moderate ☐ Intense

Experience: _____
_____
_____

Side Effects: ☐ Dry mouth ☐ Over-stimulated
☐ Drowsy ☐ Lethargic ☐ Paranoia
☐ _____

Desired Effect: ☐ Yes ☐ No ☐ _____

Rating: ★★★★★

Journal 5

Date: _____ Time: _____

Dose: _____ Method: _____

Strain/Product: _____

Last Meal: ☐ Light ☐ Moderate ☐ Heavy
When: ☐ 1 hr ☐ 2 hrs ☐ 3+ hrs

Desired effect: ☐ Pain Relief ☐ Euphoria
☐ Relaxation ☐ Reduce cravings ☐ Appetite
☐ Focus ☐ Energy ☐ Creativity ☐ Sleep
☐ _____

Pain level: _____ Stress level: _____

```
0   1   2   3   4   5   6   7   8   9   10
```

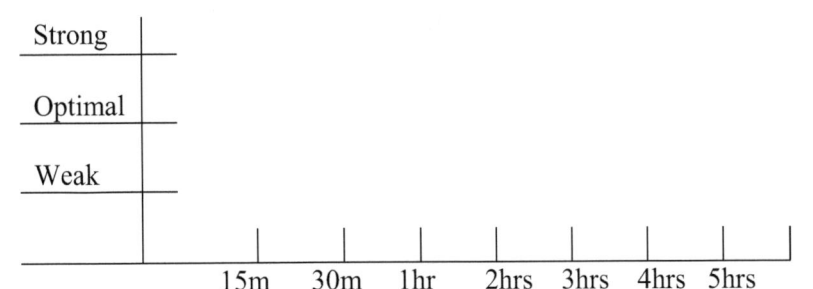

Intensity Graph:

Strong |
Optimal |
Weak |

    15m 30m 1hr 2hrs 3hrs 4hrs 5hrs

Journal 5

Phytocannabinoids Used: ☐ THCA ☐ THC
☐ THCV ☐ CBD ☐ CBG ☐ CBC ☐ CBN
☐ CBDA   ☐ _____

Terpenes Used: ☐ Humulene ☐ Limonene
☐ Pinene   ☐ Linalool   ☐ Myrcene
☐ Terpinolene ☐ Geraneol ☐ Nerolidol
☐ Ocimene ☐ Terpineol
☐ _____

Diet: ☐ Beta-caryophyllene ☐ Anti-inflammatories
☐ Pro-biotics ☐ Omegas ☐ Adaptogens
☐ Antioxidants
☐ _____

Daily Activity: ☐ Light ☐ Moderate ☐ Intense

Experience: _____
_____
_____

Side Effects: ☐ Dry mouth ☐ Over-stimulated
☐ Drowsy ☐ Lethargic ☐ Paranoia
☐ _____

Desired Effect: ☐ Yes ☐ No ☐ _____

Rating: ★★★★★

Recommended Resources

For more information on dosing and specific medical conditions aided by cannabis:
- *Cannabis Health Index* by Uwe Blesching
- *Cannabis Pharmacy: A Practical Guide to Medical Marijuana* by Michael Backes

For more information on growing cannabis:
- *Marijuana Growers Handbook* by Ed Rosenthal

For more information on crafting cannabis:
- *Edibles* by Stephanie Hua
- *The Cannabis Spa* by Sandra Hinchliffe

For more information on cannabis laws and obtaining a medical recommendation:
- www.SafeAccessNow.org

For more information on scientific research:
- National Institute of Health Online

For more information on addiction:
- *Refuge Recovery* by Noah Levine

For more information on positive thinking:
- *Power Choices* by Dr. Brenda Wade

Questions, Comments, or More Information

www.Wellness-Cannabis.com

Made in the USA
Columbia, SC
11 January 2024